BEYOND BEST PRACTICE

Written by practitioners for practitioners, this empirically grounded book offers clinicians of all backgrounds a guide to incorporating feedback and self-development strategies that will dramatically enhance their therapeutic abilities. Building on the foundation of Feedback-Informed Treatment (FIT), *Beyond Best Practice* explores the benefits of practising therapy using in-the-moment client feedback, with an emphasis on ongoing, typically solitary, *deliberate practice*.

Chapters describe the real-world journey of an established master therapist and her agency, examining each element of FIT in detail through her eyes. Her journey is illustrated through discussions with prominent researchers, authors, and former clients, as well as informative experiences outside psychotherapy. Rich case examples of success, failure, and "failing successfully" are also woven throughout, with a focus on the practical applications and skills needed to become an excellent and effective therapist and agency.

What becomes clear through the many narratives is that we can improve our services by studying the obvious and subtle forms of feedback that are available to us at all times. *Beyond Best Practice* emphasizes what each practitioner can do to become more effective, one client at a time. It will be essential reading for all mental health practitioners and agencies working at the front lines of medical care.

Birgit Valla is a Norwegian clinical psychologist and leader of a mental health service for children, families, adults, and people with addictions and substance abuse, which is developed based upon the feedback from the people seeking help. Valla is also a writer, lecturer, and public speaker.

David S. Prescott has worked in the field of treating sexual abuse for 34 years and has produced 18 book projects in the areas of abuse and psychotherapy. He lectures around the world and is the recipient of two lifetime achievement awards from international organizations. He is a senior associate for the International Center for Clinical Excellence.

"15 years from now, we will realise that we have got it wrong about a lot of things in mental health care. Birgit Valla and David Prescott point us in the direction that we need to go. They have got it right. Buy 10 copies of this book and give them to your colleagues. This book is a conversation-piece we need to have."

Daryl Chow, PhD, author of *The First Kiss: Undoing the Intake Model and Igniting First Sessions in Psychotherapy*

"This book represents ground-breaking ideas about how to think differently about mental health care all over the world. With these ideas Birgit Valla has managed to change the entire system in her home town in Norway. This book is a must-read for anybody interested in delivering better services to the people seeking help from mental health care professionals."

Susanne Bargmann, psychologist, author, trainer and international speaker, Denmark

BEYOND BEST PRACTICE

How Mental Health Services Can Be Better

Birgit Valla and David S. Prescott

Routledge
Taylor & Francis Group
LONDON AND NEW YORK

First published in English in 2019 by Routledge
2 Park Square, Milton Park, Abingdon, Oxon OX14 4RN

and by Routledge
52 Vanderbilt Avenue, New York, NY 10017

Routledge is an imprint of the Taylor & Francis Group, an informa business

Published in Norwegian by Gyldendal Norsk Forlag 2014

British Library Cataloguing-in-Publication Data
A catalogue record for this book is available from the British Library

Library of Congress Cataloging-in-Publication Data
A catalog record has been requested for this book

ISBN: 978-0-367-17510-8 (hbk)
ISBN: 978-0-367-17513-9 (pbk)
ISBN: 978-0-429-05728-1 (ebk)

Typeset in Bembo
by Swales & Willis, Exeter, Devon, UK

From Birgit: For my mother, Lise Valla, who taught me about courage.

From David: For my family, who have taught me about optimism.

CONTENTS

FOREWORD BY SCOTT D. MILLER: COMING BACK FROM THE DEAD

In 1994, Donald Miller, Jr., of the small Midwest town of Findlay, Ohio, died. His wife, Robin, did her best to move on with her life, using the federal welfare benefits available for taking care of herself and the couple's two children. Life had not been easy for the family. In the 1980s, Mr Miller fell on hard times. He lost his job and started drinking, labelling himself an "alcoholic". The couple eventually divorced. At the time of his death, he owed more than $32,000 in child support payments.

As sad as the story may be, it is all too familiar to anyone who works in the field of mental health. Life is full of difficulties, challenges, and tragedies. No sooner does one come to our attention than it is replaced by another situation equally sad or worse.

For all that, the Millers would not be so easily forgotten. Their story resurfaced in Judge Allan Davis's Hancock County Probate Court in October 2013. Present at the proceedings, besides the judge, was Mrs Miller and her very-much-alive ex-husband, Donald. As it turns out, the announcement of his death had been premature. At the time of his disappearance, acting under the extreme pressures of mood and circumstance, Mr Miller had simply jumped ship and left town. He took up residence in Florida and Georgia.

Years later, when he returned to his home town, his parents informed him he been declared dead. After failing to send word to his family about what he was doing and his whereabouts, the courts had made this determination at the request of Mrs Miller.

Seated in the courtroom, Donald soon found it was far easier to be dead than to return to the living.

"We've got the obvious here," said the judge. "A man sitting in the courtroom. He appears to be in good health."

The problem, Judge Davis asserted, was that Miller had been "dead" for nine years, thus exceeding the time limit for changing the court's prior ruling.

"It's a strange, strange situation," the Honorable Allan Davis concluded, "but as far as the law is concerned, you're still deceased."

Strange indeed. No, actually absurd. Donald Miller is clearly alive. That fact is indisputable. No one involved in the saga disagrees. And yet, for all intents and purposes, dead he remains. Rules replaced reality. Process trumped proof.

As remote as this story may seem, in reality, professional mental health finds itself in an equally absurd place. The need for help is obvious. As Mr Miller went to court to solve a problem, every day clients present for treatment to rectify a wrong, improve their lives, get a new start, feel better, and move on. To service the demand, any reasonable person would conclude that it is best to address directly, with each and every client, what they want to be different as a result of meeting with us. Instead, what happens? Year after year, massive amounts of time and money are spent defining the scope of clinical practice and standardizing service delivery. Despite our best intentions, just as in Judge Davis's court, rules ultimately replace our client's reality. Defining their problems, and regulating the methods used to treat them, trump what clients want and how best to achieve it.

As it is, 40 years of outcome research documents the futility of the field's furious, yet misplaced, efforts. While the number of standards, ethical guidelines, diagnoses, and treatment methods has exploded, almost no attention has been paid to the most important determinant of therapeutic success: client engagement. The temptation to think that the field is making huge strides in improving the quality and outcome of care is understandably strong. However, the proof is indisputable:

costs are increasing, dropout rates remain high, and overall clinical outcomes have not improved appreciably from one year to the next.

At length, clients do not care what we think about what we do or how we do it. Rather, they want what they want. And how do we figure out what is "it" that clients want? As the authors write so eloquently and convincingly in this book, *that* question is the most important of all.

I'm thrilled that this book has been revised and translated into English. The time has come to state the obvious, what everyone involved in the mental health industry already knows to be true – our clients are alive! They can and deserve to get what they want. Moreover, helpers can dramatically improve their ability to deliver the results clients seek. The old traditions have not proved their worth. It's time to set them aside and chart a new course. Brigit Valla's story shows us the way.

Scott D. Miller, Ph.D.
International Center for Clinical Excellence
Chicago, Illinois
October 2018

PREFACE BY DAVID S. PRESCOTT

A recent social media discussion for psychotherapists focused on a study by Simon Goldberg and his colleagues (2016) finding that professionals don't become more effective with experience. Outrage ensued. Examples included "I've gotten better at identifying which clients will not come back for a second session", "I'm much more effective at knowing which insurance companies will pay under what circumstances", "I can tell from the first session who will get divorced". No one talked about how they'd actually become more helpful to their clients. Even if they had, the question would have been how they had known for certain. These are the questions that a small number of practitioners began to ask many years ago.

I first met Birgit in 2013 at the Achieving Clinical Excellence conference in Amsterdam, where clinicians and researchers from around the world gathered to explore how practitioners do (and don't) improve their effectiveness. By the time of this conference, Birgit was using examples outside psychotherapy to illustrate her points about how we need feedback from our clients if we are to become better therapists. We know this implicitly. It is why some companies hire secret shoppers to test the proffered services and report on their experiences. Companies that respond to feedback earn customer loyalty. How is it that this message is so difficult to translate into psychotherapy practice?

My main inspiration for working on this book, besides Birgit herself, was in watching how practitioners in the Nordic countries from Rolf Sundet to Jakko Seikkula regarded their clients and were willing to go the extra mile to understand them. All this came at a time when meaningful case formulation has receded in many areas. In my practice, I often encounter professionals who focus on their measures more than the people they're measuring.

I've edited many publications. For years, I invited practitioners to write chapters about their work and compiled them into books. Among my hopes was always that each volume would be its own kind of conference. My plan for this project was originally to adapt an excellent book into more of a "how-to" volume and to add my own additional points along the way. Instead, I realized just how instructive this book could be on its own; a kind of illustration of what each reader can expect as they become more feedback-informed. Instead of adding to the mix and risking confusion, I put my efforts in bolstering a remarkable narrative for a wider audience.

Birgit's story, while unique in its own way, is strikingly similar to many others who have worked to become more effective with their clients. Almost all therapists want to become more effective, but as our friend Scott Miller has observed, we all too often look in the wrong places, much like the drunk who looks for his keys under the streetlight (where he can see) rather than in the dark where he lost them. The central difference in this book is that Birgit was willing to take a long hard look at our field's failings as well as then her own.

This willingness to look into a metaphorical mirror at one's own shortcomings is rare. As we explore in Chapter 5, Steve Walfish and his colleagues (Walfish, McAlister, O'Donnell, et al., 2012) found that psychotherapists almost unanimously rated themselves as more effective than their peers. One implication of this study is that we all want to become better and yet we believe we have already done so. Walfish and his colleagues showed us that viewing ourselves as being more effective than others is itself the hallmark of being average. The story in this book is one that we should aspire to: professional development as a distant shore we always sail towards.

Birgit did this alone, seeking out coaching along the way. Helping to prepare this book has provided its own form of professional development.

I hope it inspires you not only to challenge yourself, but to find others who, like Birgit, challenge you to go above and beyond your current abilities.

I am grateful to my wife, Louise, and my colleagues and supervisees who put up with my schedule during these times – Jay Wolter, Steve Tuck, Lisa D'Innocenzo, Emma Reeves, David Schwartz, and Heidi Jacobsen. A very special thanks to the original publishers at Gyldendal for making the way forward possible. I am always grateful to have had the family I did – writers all. The memories of Peter Prescott, Eleanor Lake, and Lilias and Orville Prescott were several of the stars I steered by.

PREFACE BY BIRGIT VALLA

The only person who is educated is the one who has learned how to learn and change.

— Carl Rogers

I am a psychologist and manager of Stangehelp, an easy-to-access mental health service in Stange municipality, Norway. As the leader of this service, I receive a great many suggestions from various professionals on what to do. Weekly emails come from various sources on new methods, new programmes, and new approaches that employees should be trained in, and what ideas we might implement so that we can provide high quality treatment services. So how does one choose?

Hilde was a mother I worked with because she had a troubled relationship with her teenage son. I visited them at home to observe and, to the best of my ability, provide guidance and advice. When we had been doing this for a while, interactions between the two began to work better. I became curious about what we had done that had helped. Hilde told me that "I think it turned when you commented how nice we have it here at home", a comment I had spontaneously made at one of the first visits. Hilde was a single mother and had very little money. But with good aesthetic sense she decorated her home with finds from flea markets and thrift shops. Hilde's nearest relatives had not been very supportive of her role as a mother, and she had received many negative comments from them on how she and her children lived. When the son heard that an observer like me thought they had a nice and pleasant home, he could also begin to believe that his mother was good for something. He had not heard this often earlier, and he had been hard on his mother's attempts to create a good home for him.

This commentary on what helped made me think. Was it not the advice on setting limits, or the use of appreciative attention and all the other things I had learned in textbooks, which had worked? Yes, this might have had an effect too, but it was not what appeared to be most important for Hilde. Ever since I started working as a psychologist, I have often received feedback about what is important to people that has contradicted my own preconceived assumptions.

So how do we figure out what to do in mental health services? I have struggled with the answer to this question ever since I was a graduate student. Early in my career I was lucky to learn how to start using a feedback tool in therapy, which stimulated my curiosity in every meeting with clients. As children we come into the world with an innate curiosity. Early on, I learned the word "why?" and often used it. My curiosity was soon challenged. Albert Einstein once said that it is a miracle that curiosity survives formal education. This sounded right to me. As students, it was important for us to acquire knowledge and write what we thought the examiner wanted on the test, which in turn led to high grades. We did not have much opportunity to consider whether what we were learning held up in real life. Fortunately, curiosity survived, thanks to the strong focus on feedback that I encountered in my first workplace.

I am an optimist, but as my career progressed I was often frustrated. I'm optimistic because I believe that everything is possible. I was frustrated because I met many people who felt that the help they had received had not helped them. Some also said that they had got worse. This is all too common, despite the considerable resources devoted to help. I would have thought that, with all the resources available in mental health services, it should be possible to achieve better results. Yet I often ask myself: do they really work, these things we are doing?

Luckily, I have found a way past the frustration. As leader of Stangehelp, I eventually figured out how to figure out what to do. In

Stangehelp, we are less interested in acquiring the latest methods or adopting the latest assessments, but we are very concerned about the feedback from the people we are there to help. This is not random and haphazard. In Stangehelp we do this thoroughly, consistently, and continuously. Collecting feedback is just the beginning. It's what we do with the feedback that is important for the development of good and effective services. Research on what makes some very good in their field is the basis for how we develop our service. This book addresses the concepts of feedback and deliberate practice, which we have found to be invaluable.

How do we figure out what we should do in the mental health field? When one understands this learning process, progress will follow. I hope this book will provide some reflection on how to provide mental health care and how to understand psychological problems. I hope to inspire those who want to learn and to change themselves and their service.

In working on this book, I have talked with several people in search of answers to my questions about psychology, mental health, and mental health services. You will get to know them throughout this book: they appear in one or more chapters. I am very grateful that they have taken the time to talk with me and respond to my "why?".

ACKNOWLEDGEMENTS BY BIRGIT VALLA

Nothing is created in a vacuum, and neither was this book. Since I started practising as a psychologist, I have met many people who have contributed to shaping my path and my ideas.

Thank you to Tove Huggins, the head of the Hagen Treatment Center, who took a chance on an inexperienced, recently certified psychologist. Thank you to Andy Huggins, my mentor at Hagen, and Bjørn Einar Bjørgo, an important supervisor at an early stage in my career.

Thank you to the world's best leader, Liv Langberg, operations manager at the Child and Family Welfare Service of Stange municipality, and my professional soul mate Kårhild Husom Løken, who is a mental health care adviser. You have both demonstrated great faith in and support for my professional cavorts. A thank you also goes to the management team of the Child and Family Welfare Service: Frode Guldahl, Thilla Marie Nerli Lerberg, Brit Stensrud, Vigdis Husom Gjestvang, and Leif Ove Lysgaard. A large thanks to all my fantastic colleagues who make up Stangehelp at Stange; it is all of you who give this book credibility. Thank you to the political and administrative management of Stange who have invested in Stangehelp and given us the opportunity to develop a service in accordance with the principles in this book. Last but not least: thank you to all the residents with whom we have had contact. You have taught us what it means to provide good mental health care.

Thank you also goes to Per Halvorsen, the editor of the online edition for the Norwegian Psychologists Association, who taught me how to enjoy the art of writing. Thank you to Anette Clausen, special adviser at the Norwegian Psychologists Association, for being a positive-minded discussion partner always willing to cheer me on and for having taken upon herself that task of reading the entire book at an early point in time. Thank you to all the members of the working committee for FIT at the Regional Centre for Child and Adolescent Mental Health (RBUP East and South), who have given me a solid foundation in feedback work. Thank you to Scott Miller, friend and mentor, for his supervision, inspiration, and professional confidence in the work I do as a writer, lecturer, and clinician. Thank you to Sigrun Tømmerås, who read the entire book and gave me thorough feedback. Thank you to Tobias Gustum Lindstad, who also read the book from cover to cover with a critical eye and provided suggestions for improvements.

Thank you to Ida Stendahl, my editor at Gyldendal Akademisk for the Norwegian version, who has been an enormous support throughout the entire project and offered valuable feedback. Thank you to David Prescott for doing a tremendous effort in making the book see the light of day in English.

Thank you to my big sister and important role model as a writer, Kristin Valla, who has guided me in all my writing projects, including this book. Thank you to my father, Ørnulf Valla, an inestimable partner for shared reflection and a wise member of society. Thank you to Gard, for support throughout the whole process. And thank you to my three children, Sigurd, Astrid, and Lise, my constant reminders of the most important things in life.

1

HOW EFFECTIVE ARE WE REALLY?

In all affairs, it's a healthy thing now and then to hang a question mark on the things you have long taken for granted.

Bertrand Russell

One afternoon in late August 1999, I received a phone call from the Department of Psychology at the Norwegian University of Science and Technology (NTNU). The semester was already a few days underway when it turned out that a place had opened up in the psychology programme. The woman on the phone informed me that I was the next person on the waiting list. I was thus offered a place in the programme. Delighted about the news, I called relatives in Trondheim to help me find a place to live, packed the essentials, and a few days later turned up as the last candidate for my first day in the psychology programme I had been longing to attend. And I loved being a psychology student. I attended lectures faithfully, enjoyed studying in the reading room, and got involved in student government. I devoured psychology theories in huge gulps. This was exciting material.

The last part of the programme also included supervised professional training. We would now have actual clients to test our skills. As a part of my practical training with children, I worked with a young boy accompanied by his mother. I read up on different therapeutic approaches for children and tried to follow the most appropriate method to the best of my abilities. With a supervisor and three fellow students monitoring everything I did from behind a one-way mirror, I was certain that the therapy was carried out in the best possible way. After every session, we discussed the therapy in a tutorial. I received good feedback on my relationship with the boy and everything of interest that emerged in our sessions. His statements were analysed in light of the issue in question along with my interventions as a therapist. The boy's mother sometimes attended the sessions, while on other occasions she sat in the waiting room. The therapy was carried out as prescribed, the boy and his mother seemed satisfied, and eventually we approached the final session. As a conclusion to the therapy, I had a session with the mother to sum up and ask her about how she had experienced the contact. It was now early summer, so my supervisor and two of my fellow students were away on holiday. However, I did not consider this to be a problem; up to that point I had had many sessions with the mother and boy and felt relatively secure about our relationship. Only one fellow student remained to sit behind the mirror and give me feedback afterwards.

The mother arrived for our appointment and on this occasion had brought along her live-in partner, whom I had not met before. She seemed a bit uncomfortable and I asked her how she thought the therapy had been. She replied that it hadn't been in any sense as she'd expected. On the contrary, she was quite disappointed with all of it, and did not think it had helped very much with the boy's problems. She'd had completely different expectations for the help they would receive and described what she had envisioned. It turned out that she had very clear ideas. I listened to her feedback, resisted the need to defend myself, and hoped that I demonstrated understanding for her experience. We then ended the session and said our goodbyes. Demoralized, I went to join the one fellow student who had witnessed the entire episode to collect myself. "You could not have received such negative feedback in a better way," she said in consolation, trying to restore my confidence.

Over the years since then, I have often thought that I would like to be able to thank the mother. To this day, I appreciate her giving me excellent feedback at such an early stage in my career on what I was doing that was ineffective. In many ways, it has shaped me as a psychologist.

In both my university education and later, when taking part in different courses and specialized studies, there was little focus on integrating the ideas of the client with the therapist's knowledge when it came to determining what should be done in therapy. The phrase "client participation" has of course been used frequently, but the opinions of the client have come second or as an afterthought to what the therapist believes to be best – if one even remembers to ask. Ever since I was a student, I have been interested in understanding how I can find the best way to work with a given client, with a basis in my expertise as a therapist. I have discovered that the process that I was taught to use for determining this contains serious drawbacks, and I have therefore searched for another way to determine how to help people who are struggling with psychological problems. In 2010, I wrote an article about how clients should play a leading role in determining the design of their own treatment (Valla, 2010). Since that time, I have developed these ideas further, and I believe that the process by which we determine what we will do to help people should be quite different from the traditional practice, which is also established in structures and legislation within the field of mental health care. For many people, my thoughts are probably not new. When you read this book you might discover that you are already working this way.

There are good reasons for starting to think differently within the field of mental health care. The first chapter addresses this book's point of departure: therapy works, but perhaps not as well as we would like to believe. There is clearly room for improvement.

Therapy works

The experience from my studies stands in stark contrast to the experiences of my childhood. I come from a small town in Nordland county, Norway, with a population of around 400. Just before the Second World War, my grandfather built the house where I grew up, a large villa in the timely style of functionalism. My mother was born and raised in Oslo, but as a recently licensed psychologist, she moved to Northern Norway to get away from the academic community and learn how to "talk to the people in the countryside", as she put it. There she met my father and they moved into my grandfather's big house.

When I was a little girl, my mother's private practice was in the basement. She viewed this as being practical, because in this way she was always at home and close to her children, even though she was busy with her clients. There weren't many psychologists in these parts and for that reason people travelled from far and wide to see my mother. I never really understood what they were doing behind the soundproof door to what we called the treatment room, but I knew it was supposed to help people who were not feeling well. Sometimes they brought along their children and then I would play with them while their mothers were talking to my mother. These people seemed to get better, because I noticed that they thanked my mother and were pleased about the contact they had with her. Since she died, I have met people who have expressed to me how much the help she gave them has meant to them. I have, in other words, grown up with a belief that therapy works.

My childhood experiences were wholly correct. That therapy is often effective has been scientifically proven. Viewed from a historical perspective, it has been important to demonstrate that psychotherapy actually works. In the 1950s and 1960s, the research scientist Hans Eysenck claimed in a number of articles that psychotherapy is not effective and that it could even be harmful (Eysenck, 1957, 1966). Eysenck defined psychotherapy as psychodynamic and eclectic approaches, but behavioural therapy, of which he was an adherent, was something different. In the years following the publication of Eysenck's claims, two fronts emerged: one advocated behavioural therapeutic approaches, while research scientists like Saul Rosenzweig (1936), Allen Bergin (1978), and Lester Luborsky (1954; Luborsky, Singer, & Luborsky, 1975) defended more traditional psychotherapy.

It wasn't until 1977 that Mary Lee Smith and Gene Glass intervened with an alternative method for examining the effect of psychotherapy, specifically meta-analysis. As a research strategy, instead of carrying out new research on new subjects, meta-analysis entails analysing the results of previous studies. Smith and Glass's (1977) first article, "Meta-analysis of psychotherapy outcome studies", was groundbreaking research that drew attention from all over the world. They found that psychotherapy was extremely effective as a treatment approach, and the debate was dramatically changed. Today their study is considered to be one of "40 studies that changed psychology" and remains one of the most frequently cited studies within psychology. Since Smith and Glass's first study, a large number of other studies have shown that psychotherapy is an effective form of treatment. This is now a well-established finding. Meta-analysis has determined that psychotherapy has an effect size of 0.8 (Wampold, 2001), which means that 80% of those who complete treatment experience more improvement than those who do not receive treatment. This is considered an extremely large effect size, and we have good reason to pat ourselves on the back when it comes to psychotherapy as a treatment approach. But what does that mean, really? I will return to this later.

Another means of assessing the impact of psychotherapy is through something called "numbers needed to treat" (NNT), which refers to how many people must be treated to achieve an effect. For psychotherapy this is the number 3. In other words, you must treat three people in order to be able to say that the mental health of one person has improved. This perhaps does not sound very promising, but let us look at other treatment forms that many people view as being very effective. For the flu vaccine, the number is 12. For the treatment of acute asthma, it is 9. The number for aspirin as a heart attack prevention measure is 176. I can also add that lice shampoo as a treatment for children with head lice is very effective. The number is two.

Some history of psychology and psychological problems

Let's take a quick look back in time. We introduced this book by stating that psychotherapy can be effective. It is the prevailing method for helping people with psychological problems, but psychotherapy has also evolved in keeping with the way in which we understand psychological problems. The process of psychotherapy can entail a variety of approaches and as a treatment form is far from uniform. The evolution of psychotherapy and the understanding of psychological problems must be viewed in the context of the development of the field of psychology and in light of the greater culture and society.

Volda University College professor Tor Johan Ekeland knows a lot about the history of psychology. I have been reading his articles ever since my student days, and his critical perspective on the profession has been inspiring. After reading his most recent article in the Journal of the Norwegian Psychological Association (Ekeland, 2012), I decided to call him for an in-depth chat. What interests me in particular is his description of the two cultures of psychology. In a classic essay from 1959, the scientist C.P. Snow (2001) addressed the relation between the cultures of the natural sciences and the humanities. The sciences have the ambition of being able to *explain* behaviour with an eye towards *prediction* and *control.* The humanities' ambition is *understanding,* in other words investigating how we interpret the world around us.

I asked Ekeland how these two cultures have impacted psychology.

> Psychology includes both these cultures, that is what makes the discipline unwieldy. The foundation of our discipline contains a knowledge-based opposition that is the source of a lot of conflict, and the research communities have not succeeded in handling this opposition. The dominant culture in the research communities has varied. In the early 1970s, psychology was defined as a social science, and at universities psychology has often been categorized as belonging to the social sciences. But in some places psychology is situated in the faculty of medicine and there it has greater prestige.

I asked Ekeland whether one of the cultures has a higher status than the other. "Yes, obviously," he said, "and there is no doubt that it is the natural science culture that has constituted the basis for psychology's development and identity." According to Ekeland, the result of this has been that a lot of research in psychology is about individuals, but little about *people*; a lot about behaviour, but little about *actions*; a lot about emotional states, but little about *subjectivity*; a lot about cognition, but little about *meaning*; a lot about responses and reactions, but little about *intentions and human beings' self-determination.*

I asked him what has influenced the orientation of psychology's evolution. Ekeland mentioned social changes that have taken place outside of psychology but that nonetheless influence it.

> Psychology has always been a weak discipline from a purely scientific standpoint, given the strong oppositions between the two cultures it has struggled with. It has, therefore, been easily influenced by fluctuations in society at large. In the 1970s, psychology emerged as a social science in opposition to what it had been previously when physics and behavioural psychology dominated. Then came the computer revolution, and the cognitive perspective acquired broad prominence. Now it is the revolution of the brain that prevails. We have acquired new technology to study the brain and this gives us new opportunities for understanding the human being. Over the course of these decades, society has become more and more individualistic and individual-orientated, and the perspective on the interaction between the individual and society has been undermined. And psychology follows suit.

Ekeland also explained that psychiatry has played a critical role in determining how psychologists carry out their work. In the 1970s, a scathing critique of psychiatry emerged, primarily targeting the institutional psychiatry that prevailed in the 1950s and 1960s. This resulted in a dismantling of the institutions, and it was believed that it would also lead to a curtailment of the medical understanding. However, that did not come to pass. Psychiatry began a reorientation. Its identity had previously been in the institutions and was now concerned about rebuilding confidence. It was thus a matter of reinforcing the scientific foundation and returning to the natural sciences. This found expression through a power struggle in the American Psychiatric Association, which culminated in a revision of the American system for diagnosis (American Psychiatric Association, 1980), entailing a return to a fundamentally biological model. There was a simultaneous increase in the number of diagnoses.

"Diagnoses have been of great importance for the discipline of psychiatry," Ekeland stated,

> and they have changed. After WWII, the diagnoses within psychiatry had a low status for professional reasons. It was psychodynamic thought that prevailed, and problems were interpreted as an expression of something having to do with a person's life history and context. A diagnosis was not interesting in terms of understanding the problem. The thinking was more in keeping with the culture of the humanities. In the 1970s and 1980s, this was turned around. The

> diagnosis manual and its adherents acquired great power and influence with respect to how the field developed in the years to come. It turned out to be much simpler to sell individual diagnostics than contextual perspectives.

Ekeland was concerned about the fact that it is the medical model that predominates within the mental health care services.

> This is a part of the culture of the natural sciences, and researchers and professionals are interested in developing knowledge about treatment that can tell us if one applies a specific method to a defined problem, one will achieve a given outcome. The diagnoses are used as a basis for determining the type of treatment to be offered and they are based on a cause and effect connection. The public authorities impose strict requirements for professional practice and documentation and professionals are to use methods based on research findings. The concept of evidence has become the prevailing stamp of quality within service provision, and it is a matter of determining "what" works, so the professions employ the correct psychotherapeutic knowledge. The problem with this approach to mental health care is that such a stable connection does not exist in psychotherapy. In the relevant research, there is little support for the diagnoses in and of themselves. Diagnosing is supposed to help us clarify and provide a better understanding of the problem, but this is contingent upon the diagnostics being valid; in other words, that diagnostics can establish the existence of illnesses and predict which treatment is the best. While somatic illnesses can for the most part be demonstrated objectively, psychiatric diagnoses are constructions; they refer to social data (thoughts, feelings, and behaviour) and are based on a consensus within the discipline about what it means to be sick or healthy. The diagnosis in itself only offers a weak indication of what the treatment should be, quite simply because it does not say anything about the patient as a person and subject. One can put it like this: In this field, one cannot treat illnesses the way one understands this in a somatic sense, one can only treat "sick" people. In short, this is precisely what many decades of treatment research prove. This means that psychotherapy as a treatment form for psychological problems will never be able to work in the same way as treatment forms for somatic illnesses. Mental health care must therefore be provided on the basis of the other culture, the humanities, in which the context and subject play a part to a much greater extent.

Psychotherapeutic methods have experienced formidable growth in the last few decades, which has also been positive in terms of providing therapists with more methods for helping people with psychological problems. However, there has been little focus on the more negative aspects of therapy, and we will therefore return to the world of therapy and look at its problematic aspects.

When therapy is harmful

Michael Lambert is a professor of psychology at Brigham Young University in the USA. He is a pioneer in research on psychotherapy and is particularly well known for his interest in finding out what leads to change in therapy. He is perhaps less well known for his interest in the more negative aspects of therapy, which he began researching while he was still a PhD candidate. Becoming curious about Lambert's research, I decided to make a telephone appointment with him. We started the conversation by speaking about precisely these negative aspects. Early in his career Lambert, together with the researchers Allen Bergin and J.L. Collins, wrote a chapter about the negative effects of therapy and how the therapist contributes to therapy, aggravating problems in some patients (Lambert, Bergin, & Collins, 1977).

I asked Lambert if this chapter received a lot of attention. "No, unfortunately not," he answered. "It is a very good chapter, and I don't think anyone has done such a thorough job on the subject, even today. It's just a shame that nobody read it, and it did not have much influence on the discipline."

I had not heard about the chapter either before Lambert told me about it. He sent it to me by email and I read it with great interest. Identifying clients whose conditions are aggravated by therapy and then seeking to learn from this is a subject that has been overlooked. His chapter also emphasizes how some therapists are very effective, while others achieve generally poor results. In my education, there had been little importance attributed to whether I as a therapist might contribute to a poor outcome. On the contrary, I remember that one of my supervisors from my professional training told us that psychologists are seldom the cause of unfortunate therapeutic outcomes. I need not worry about that; this was almost always due to something in the client. So, we analysed the client's thoughts, feelings, and actions in the tutorials. This puzzled me, even at that time. Since concluding my training, I have been interested in precisely the contribution of therapists to the outcome of therapy.

One person who has experienced how harmful therapy can be is Sigrun Tømmerås. Tømmerås was a guest writer for the *Journal of the Norwegian Psychological Association* in 2010 and contributed the article "Når terapien skader" ("When therapy is harmful"), in which she told of her experiences as a client. I have also become acquainted with her through her blog and her activity on Twitter. I have always recognized her as an intelligent woman, and I called her to learn more about the experience of therapy from the position of the client.

Tømmerås tells me about the psychologist with a private practice whom she saw for four years, a therapeutic process that had enormously negative consequences. She experienced the therapist as being quite authoritarian and did not receive help with issues she initially had sought out therapy to address, specifically, processing childhood traumas. Tømmerås's experience was that the psychologist's understanding occupied almost all the space in the therapy situation, and she started doubting herself and her own experiences. She believed that it was perhaps she who had misunderstood or had the wrong expectations and that her thoughts were abnormal. Eventually she completely lost the ability to express herself. She still finds it difficult to explain why this occurred, but it was as if her own expression had been shut down. After concluding the therapy, she went through a long period during which she was completely numb and apathetic. She had nightmares about the therapist and lost the ability to feel anything, including hunger or thirst. She told me that it was the most painful thing she had experienced in her adult life. She became incredibly lonely in this numbness and did not know of anyone else who had experienced such a thing.

"It didn't seem as if he noticed that he had traumatized me," she told me:

> When I spoke with him on the telephone about it afterwards, he said that he couldn't see that there was anything he could have done differently. But in the journal, he describes me as much worse when I left than when I began, so I don't understand how he can be satisfied with the job he did.

Tømmerås concluded her therapy in 2001; she couldn't take any more. At the time, she felt quite blunted emotionally, but she talked about it a great deal and had a compelling need to tell others about her experiences. At a seminar, she met another participant who was extremely critical of mental health care, and they stayed in touch. They inspired one another, and when she read a feature article in the national daily *Dagbladet* about diagnoses it served as a catalyst, and she found the courage to write a response. *Dagbladet* printed her response, which was the beginning of a long series of newspaper segments in both local and national newspapers.

> It is perhaps a bit of an exaggeration, but it was like therapy for me. Starting to write was a big step; it was a way of coming to grips with the experiences. The numbness gradually disappeared, and I began to find myself again. I experienced having been so incapacitated and pathologized by the therapy, so the fact that newspapers printed my articles without giving me a diagnosis was like being given a clean bill of health. In the therapy setting, my experience was that I could say things that were given a negative interpretation. When I said the same thing in another context, such as in a newspaper article, I was met with positive interest.

Tømmerås is not alone in having had such experiences from therapy. Ever since I finished my studies, I have read about such experiences on blogs and heard stories from people I have met. I have had a lot of contact with client organizations and former clients of mental health care services, from whom I have learned what has been useful and what has been harmful. Some of the stories have been upsetting and profoundly moving. That was how it was when I met Guro.

Guro grew up with her mother, father, and two brothers in a medium-sized village in Norway. She describes her childhood as being quite normal. She received a lot of love and care at home and views the first years of her life as having been secure and good. However, Guro was also a sensitive child, and her schooling introduced some insecurities that came to a head when she started college. At the age of 18, she was put on antidepressants for the first time, which would prove to have serious consequences for her in the years that followed. For three or four years, she took a small dose of the medication. After a traumatic experience at the age of 22, the dosage was increased, and Guro had a strong reaction to this. Her anxiety increased, she became dizzy and felt worse than ever before. Finally, Guro had to be institutionalized in a psychiatric hospital. There, the medication prescribed increased dramatically. Guro tells of the experience of the hospital,

> I thought I was crazy. It felt like I was inside a strange, frightening world, and I had many bizarre thoughts. I experienced anxiety, withdrawal symptoms and tried frantically to explain to the doctors and nurses what was happening to me. I tore at my hair, it felt like electric currents were running from my head and down into my body. It was like being in a horror film, as if I had come to hell on earth. It destroyed a great deal of my life. The diagnosis they gave me was personality disorder. I received a cocktail of medication that had enormous side effects and produced withdrawal symptoms. What happened to me was caused by the medication, not a personality disorder!

Today, Guro is not taking any medication, but the tensions have lodged themselves in her body and are the source of great physical pain. She still has nightmares about what happened when she was institutionalized. The traumas still have a hold on her, despite many discussions about what happened. However, Guro is optimistic and refuses to allow the events destroy the rest of her life. She says, "Inside me there are many things that I love! Being in the outdoors, being with friends. I love life, after all!"

I wish I could say that Guro's story was unique, but it is unfortunately just one of many. Some of the stories had less serious consequences, while others are accounts of seriously reduced quality of life and long-term damage in the wake of treatment. Are we actually as effective as we like to believe?

I explained my scepticism about the impact of therapy to Michael Lambert and asked him how effective we actually are in ordinary clinical practice. Lambert told me that this effect size of 0.8 comes from what are called clinical trials, for which the clients are carefully handpicked to match the criteria of a specific problem. Then they receive relatively extensive treatment (12–14 weeks) by therapists who are assessed on their results and under supervision. In such a context, 40 to 60 or 70% will experience some kind of recovery. In a clinical context, such results will potentially be repeated if the conditions are the same. However, if one looks at what constitutes standard health care in the USA, the figures are not nearly as good. Then it is closer to a third of clients who experience an improvement, and they do not receive as extensive treatment, not by far. There are, of course, variations between treatment contexts. If the treatment is more thorough, the results also go up.

I asked him: what about those who drop out? Are they included in this 0.8 effect size? Lambert said that usually these individuals are replaced, so they are not included.

> One has to read the research articles carefully. When one is going to analyse data, one is speaking about one selection of data that is called "with the intention of being treated" and another selection called "completed". When it comes to the 0.8 effect size, we are speaking about the "completed" selection.

"Actually," Lambert said, "the results from ordinary clinical practice are quite alarming."

So, my concerns about the effectiveness of therapy have not been wholly groundless.

Help that works

When I had completed my studies in January 2005, my question was: is this really the best we can do? I thought I had done everything correctly in my treatment with the boy during my studies, based on what I had learned. All the same, the outcome was discouraging. Since that time, my answer has been a definitive no. For nine years, I have systematically requested feedback from every single person I have met in therapy on what has been effective for them and how they experienced the encounter with me. I have worked in specialist health services and in the public sector, with children and adults, and with many different issues. What strikes me is that those of us working in mental health care services do a lot of things that, according to many people, have very little significance. I have also found that we do too little of what many people view as very important and which often has to do with life experience. We should do more of what the clients think is important and less of everything else. In order to succeed in doing so, we must listen to those we are trying to help in order to determine what is what.

All the years I have spent collecting feedback from users have led to many thoughts about how we should develop mental health care services for the future. I have concluded that it is possible to provide far more effective and competent help than what is currently being offered through mental health care services. However, that would require us to recognize that the services must be changed, and to have the will and courage to move in another direction. This book is an idea of how we can begin to move this work forward. The basis for the development of mental health care services should be feedback from those who receive them and what they experience as useful. Within the field of mental health care, we have been interested in such feedback far too little, especially when it has contradicted the prevailing conceptual paradigm.

The next chapter looks at the foundation of knowledge on which the development of mental health care services is based and demonstrates how we can expand our understanding of what constitutes relevant knowledge. I will address in further detail what it means to acquire feedback from those we are helping, and then, in Chapter 4, explain how we can use this feedback to bring about recovery. Chapter 5 addresses how we can develop as individual therapists. Chapter 6 tells how organizations can develop in response to feedback on what helps. I will then address the obvious feedback clients give us all the time, if only we will open our minds and accept it. Finally, I will say something about the road ahead for mental health care services of the future.

2

KNOWLEDGE

How can we remember our ignorance, which our growth requires, when we are using our knowledge all the time?

Henry David Thoreau

Round bales

While I was still a student, I had a young client who had quite a long drive when he came to see me. He did not live in the city of Trondheim, but a substantial distance away in the countryside. Once when he came to see me he wanted to tell me something about his father (and as a psychologist I am always interested in the relationship between father and son, especially when it is problematic in nature). In the middle of the story, which was about a field and a tractor, he started talking about something he called *roinballa*. I didn't understand this at all and made a few attempts to clarify what he was talking about. Finally, the boy realized that I didn't understand him and returned to the topic we had been talking about before he got sidetracked with his story.

In my subsequent tutorial, fortunately for me, one of my fellow students was from Trondheim and had grown up in a rural area. She was able to explain to me that *roinballa* (a dialect derivation of the Norwegian word *rundballer*) are round bales of hay, the kind one sometimes sees scattered across the fields. The boy had been trying to tell me something related to these round bales, something he'd done with his father. I don't remember much from that particular therapy, but I remember the "round bales" and the feeling that I was missing out on something crucial from this boy's world.

Knowledge comes in many forms. One can read a book or an article, or one can learn by practising methods. Still, our methods and knowledge are not particularly helpful if they are not a good fit with the experiences of those we meet. This is what makes it all complicated, demanding, exciting, and educational. We don't know ahead of time what is a good fit for each person. We have to figure this out in collaboration with each individual, as we get to know them.

I am quite certain that knowledge helps. The more I know about a given subject, the better able I will be to develop a nuanced approach, and the better I know a local community, the more prepared I will be to help. But this alone isn't enough. We must also use our head and heart. One of my clients wrote me the following words: "You are sincere, and you are genuine, and you are a little bit strict, and it is completely appropriate for you to be so. But you are so kind and good and friendly. You emanate an infectious feeling of peace." This kind of quality cannot be learned from a book.

In this chapter I will explore the type of knowledge we need to be good helpers. A lot of research has been done on what is effective in therapy. Here the experts have difficulties reaching a consensus. A lot of psychotherapy research has explored various methods in the effort to determine which approaches might be best suited for different sets of problems. I have attempted to show how the conditions for this type of research should probably be changed. We have a great deal of other kinds of knowledge that is much more important than rote methods, and that is something that will be gradually illuminated as throughout this chapter. Finally, the knowledge you gain from the person you are supposed to help is the most important: this individual's understanding of his or her life. This is knowledge you can't get from reading up on it. This is knowledge you find in the moment. If you pay attention to this information, you will learn something new every day.

Psychotherapy research

The question of what is effective in therapy has been the subject of research and discussion since therapy's origins. As far back as in 1936, Saul Rosenzweig suggested that there were factors that all forms of therapy shared which were the effective elements, also known as "common factors". With his article "Some implicit common factors in diverse methods of psychotherapy" he was the first to put into words the now well-known dodo bird verdict within psychotherapy. This is taken from Lewis Carroll's novel *Alice in Wonderland* and refers to the race the dodo bird arranged so everyone would be dry after having swum around in Alice's tears. The dodo bird designed a racetrack, like a kind of ring, and then he lined up participants along a line, some here and others there. When they all began to run when they felt like it and stop when they felt like it, understanding when the race was over was no easy matter. They had been running for about half an hour and were dry again when the dodo bird proclaimed: "The race is over!" When they wanted to know who had won, he had to think about it for a while before he said, "Everybody has won and all must have prizes." That applies to psychotherapeutic methods as well, Rosenzweig claimed. None of the methods appears to be better than others; they are effective because of what they have in common.

Since that time, there has been a formidable research investment focused on finding evidence to demonstrate that some methods are, in fact, more effective for specific ailments than others. Particularly within cognitive therapy or similar types of therapy, there has been a lot of interest in this research. In a typical research design, the method in question has been compared with traditional therapy, specialized counselling or a control group (e.g. people on a waiting list). Parallel to this, the research shows that it is not specific ingredients that are effective in a particular therapy, but rather what the therapy forms have in common. Over time, the opinion that no particular therapy method stands above the rest has garnered considerable support.

Bruce Wampold has done a lot of research on this topic. Initially a mathematician, he later earned a PhD in psychology and has written many research articles on the subject of psychotherapy. He is perhaps best known for the book *The Great Psychotherapy Debate* (2001), a summary and analysis of therapeutic research up to that time. I met Wampold for the first time in Oslo in 2005. At the time, I had only been working as a psychologist for a few months but had already begun to see that the knowledge I had acquired through my studies was not always applicable to human beings in real life. Although what I had learned was enormously useful, it seemed that I continually had to adapt the knowledge, combine it in different ways, or think completely differently. This meant working in cooperation with the families and helping them by starting with their own ideas. Wampold's lecture made an impression on me. In the years that followed, I have had the opportunity to talk to him both in the USA and in Hamar, Norway, and corresponded with him by email regarding questions about psychotherapy research. After I started writing this book, however, I became aware that I needed to have an in-depth conversation with him in order to adequately get to the bottom of the psychotherapy issue. Wampold had by that time been appointed head of research at the Modum Bad Psychiatric Center in Buskerud and visited Norway often. I had the chance to schedule a meeting with him on a spring day in 2012.

Modum is a beautiful place. I met Wampold at the research centre and while he was finishing up for the day with his doctoral students I looked around the building. In the stairway leading up to the second floor there were photographs of researchers and students hanging on the walls and all the PhD diplomas had been framed. Wampold and I strolled down to the little cabin where he lives when he is in Norway. The Modum Bad institute consists of many buildings, many of which were built as a health spa and resort in the 19th century. Today, Modum offers a wide range of services and accepts patients from all over Norway.

With a tape recorder between us and a cup of tea in my hand, I started on my questions. The first thing I wanted to know was how Wampold became interested in psychotherapy research and what was decisive in determining the direction he chose. Wampold told me about the time he was teaching psychology at a university in the early 1990s. He used to teach his students that for some ailments there are certain treatment forms that are better than others, and the students had to learn what these were. Then he taught a course about psychotherapy research. As a reading assignment he gave the students a chapter from *The Handbook of Psychotherapy and Behavior Change* (Orlinsky, Rønnestad, & Willutzki, 2004) and the original research this chapter was based on. Wampold challenged them to determine whether the conclusion arrived at in the chapter was substantiated. The students did the assignment and returned with the following response: "This chapter says that behavioral therapy is the best form of treatment, but when we read the research behind it, we don't really think that it supports the conclusion." Wampold asked to see the research and it turned out that the students were right, with respect to not just behavioural therapy but many other forms of therapy as well. Together with the students, he decided to do his own research.

Wampold told me that this discovery upset him in two ways.

> First of all it upset me as a researcher. The idea is that we are supposed to interpret the research honestly, and I don't think this was an objective interpretation. Secondly, it upset me that they made recommendations for the types of treatments users should receive, which were not based on evidence from the research. This limits the patients' treatment options. The therapists were also told that they could only use one type of treatment and not another.

That was how it began. We moved on to talk about randomized clinical trials (RCT) studies. When a study is randomized it means that the treatment a patient receives is random (for example, determined by drawing lots). In the simplest of terms, randomized clinical studies on methods within psychotherapy are done as follows: one wants to determine the effectiveness of a method for a specific problem. One then creates a design whereby a group of patients who receive treatment using the method in question is compared with a control group, often referred to as "TAU" (treatment as usual). In other words, the control group receives the type of therapy as is ordinarily provided in daily clinical practice. In some cases, this means that the TAU is less structured and not conducted as diligently as the method under study. In such studies, the method in question almost always does better than the control group. There is then a very strong question as to whether it really is the method that is the determining factor.

There were a number of problems with these studies. Actually, there were so many problems that Wampold was not sure where to begin. First of all, the study is not double-blinded, as is standard within the field of medicine. In medicine, when a patient in a study receives medicine or a placebo, the person administering the medication does not know which pill it is. In RCT studies of psychotherapy, the therapist knows that he or she is giving the control group treatment (and may have strong opinions about being in the treatment or control conditions), and the client can figure this out quickly. Second, the treatments within medicine look the same, while in psychotherapy they are extremely different, and many subtle manipulations occur in the control treatment context. Third, the person providing the treatment is not taken into consideration; they are not just any therapists. The therapists being studied receive training and guidance, then assess their results. This is not something that takes place in ordinary clinical practice. And worse yet: the study ignores the therapist effect (the fact that some therapists achieve much better results than others). Even in clinical studies there are some therapists who have better outcomes than others. Under these conditions, it is not surprising when the treatment method under study functions very well. The problem is that the methods in question are probably no more or less effective than other approaches employed under equivalent conditions. In studies comparing two or more bona fide methods under identical conditions, usually there is no difference in the results. A fundamental question for all people reading this research to ask is "what kind of treatment are they actually comparing their method to?".

Treatment methods have also proven to constitute only a small part of what is effective in therapy. More important factors include the choice of therapist, the alliance between client and therapist, providing treatment within the strong personal values of the client, and whether the client believes the therapy will help. Research suggests that methods have little or no importance, but it's not that simple. Methods can be an important part of the alliance. The alliance, according to psychotherapy research, is about both reaching an agreement on goals (what the client wants to achieve through the therapy), agreement on a working method (how to achieve the goals, which is where method comes in) and the relational bond between client and therapist. It is important that both the client and the therapist have faith that all of this will be effective.

A plethora of methods

It is impossible to know in advance what method will best suit each client, based simply on a standard case file, as we saw in my conversation with Ekeland in Chapter 1. Nonetheless, we are overwhelmed by methods, which state guidelines that the professional community expects us to implement. I don't know how many times I have attended a course, a seminar, or a conference and been presented with a new method that was supposed to be better than anything that came before. I have even believed that finally I'd found an approach that could help me solve the issues of a particular family that were confounding me at the time. Full of enthusiasm I went home and looked forward to the next session with the family. In my head I envisioned how successful the new approach will be, and we would all be happy to finally experience doing something that helps. The reality is almost never as I envision it. Usually the families are far from as enthusiastic about my new knowledge as I am and often present more information. Often the consequence is that I realize that this will not turn out like the miracle example I heard about in training.

When I have encountered challenges with clients that made me realize I had little experience or knowledge about the problem, I have focused on the alliance with the clients as being the most important and started there. I have always been able to trust that my clients would let me know if we were on the wrong track. They have either given me feedback at the end of our session about how they experience our contact or given me feedback indicating that they feel better. If they do not experience improvement within a reasonable timeframe, I know that we are on the wrong track. Then we have discussed what would be a more appropriate procedure. Still, the clients expect me to know more than they do. They expect me to offer them something that they don't know about themselves, to contribute something extra. In the context of unknown or difficult issues I have read up on the related research and sought knowledge that I hope will be helpful the next time we meet.

Trampoline therapy

That's how it was with Eva and her son, Simen. After the experience I had during my studies, I started to ask some hard questions about how I could help the young people who came to me. I was fortunate to make the acquaintance of Eva and Simen early in my professional career. Simen was a 10-year-old boy struggling a great deal following the suicide of his brother a year before. He had witnessed many of the events surrounding his brother's suicide, which had occurred in the family home. Afterwards, he had been well cared for by his mother and other loved ones, but Simen was not a boy who found it easy to put his thoughts and feelings into words, so there was nobody who felt they could reach him. He became anxious and avoided situations that reminded him of the suicide. He sometimes had nightmares and was completely dependent on his mother most of the time. At school, he had difficulty concentrating and became introverted. Finally, Eva decided the best course of action was to send him to the children and young people's psychiatric outpatient clinic (referred to as the BUP) to receive some help. There the treatment consisted of play therapy and a sandbox. Simen did not want any part of this and had to be carried up the stairs to BUP and into the play therapy room, where he sat beside the sandbox and refused to say anything. After a few visits like this, BUP essentially gave up and referred Simen to the treatment centre where I worked.

I met Simen for the first time in his family's home, the kind of house where everyone feels welcome. The kitchen was the heart of the home, and Eva always had something tasty waiting for visitors. After a little coffee and a chat with Eva, while Simen slinked around us, sizing me up, I was finally allowed to accompany him to see his bedroom. He was an enthusiastic Lego builder, something I personally find quite fun, so we started with a common interest. When I was going to leave after the first meeting, Simen came over to me and gave me a spontaneous hug. We would soon meet again.

For my next meeting with Simen, he came to visit my place of work. There is a large gymnasium there where we spent time together. Since the first meeting, I had read up on talking with children about trauma, eagerly devouring articles by Atle Dyregrov and others on the subject. I tried implementing this material with Simen to get him to open up a little bit, but he was dismissive. He would ignore my attempts to broach the subject of the traumatic event and find something else to do. There was no hug when it was time for him and Eva to leave. I wondered about how this therapy would go.

We had agreed to meet in the gymnasium again, but a few days later Eva called me. She told me that Simen liked being with me very much but that he'd told her: "If Birgit wants to talk with me, she has to come to our house. If I am going to visit her, then I just want to play." We immediately changed the appointment to a home visit.

Over the course of that spring, I visited Simen in his home several times. Early on, Eva and I agreed that a girlfriend of hers would also be there, someone who had been with the family on the evening Simen's brother had committed suicide. She was the one who had taken care of Simen after Eva left for the hospital. We had agreed to try and talk our way through what had happened while Simen was there, but he didn't want to. First, he said that he wanted to go out and play while we talked, but I was able to persuade him to go into the room next to the kitchen, where we were sitting. I started by asking Eva and her friend relatively trivial questions, such as on which day it had happened and other ordinary things about that day. Eventually, Simen came creeping out of the room and sat on Eva's lap. He had to correct her, because her memory of the details was not perfectly accurate. For the rest of the conversation he sat completely still while Eva and her friend told me what had happened. I asked questions drawing from the knowledge I had acquired through my studies about the treatment of trauma and both Eva and her friend intermittently cried and smiled. Simen scarcely uttered a sound throughout the entire conversation. The only thing he said was: "You're crying, Mommy." Eva had been very careful to hide her tears from Simen, something she later told me perhaps had not been such a good idea.

After this, Simen's symptoms gradually began to disappear. He still didn't talk much, but he was more light-hearted and not as anxious as he'd been before. We also did other things together that were related to his brother, such as visit his grave. Then one day, Eva called and told me that I had to come, because they had decided to set up the trampoline again. Simen's big brother had been a trampoline champion and had spent a lot of time jumping on it with Simen. After his death they couldn't bring themselves to set it up. Now they were ready, and they wanted me to be there. When I arrived, Eva and Simen were well under way with the assembly process. I helped to attach the mat and the safety net. When we'd finished, Simen and I climbed up onto the trampoline and jumped on it together. With a big smile on his face, Simen told me about his big brother, who could do somersaults both forwards and backwards and who jumped higher than anyone else. I thought then that we had now completed the therapy process.

One of the compulsory requirements for becoming a specialist in clinical child and adolescent psychology is 240 hours of practice under the supervision of psychology specialists, a requirement which I eventually completed. However, Simen and Eva were among the best instructors I had. On my own, I wouldn't have had the imagination to come up with everything we did together. They told me at an early stage of our contact what was important for Simen. When they discovered that I took their feedback seriously, they started giving me more input on what Simen needed to feel better. They appreciated that I allowed them to guide me.

Evidence-based?

But how can we know whether we are employing the proper therapeutic techniques? If we can only use methods on which RCT studies have been done, our therapeutic resources will be scant. I ask Wampold about this. He said that it is not the method that should be subjected to a standard, but the therapist. The therapist can apply any method they choose as long as it is ethically sound and has a meaningful substantiation: as long as it works.

The problem with rote methods is all the times they don't work. When one has worked as a therapist for a while, one sees this happens often enough. There are times and cases to do things a bit differently, a bit through trial and error, and perhaps in collaboration with the client arrive at something completely new. The next question was whether this could be as effective as the methods backed up by countless RCT studies. During my meeting with Wampold I suggested this idea to him and asked:

> So imagine, I invent a method or therapeutic approach that has a reasonable basis and that both the client and I think it is sensible to follow. If I find somebody willing to invest a lot of money to compare this method with a group that is not receiving any special type of treatment [in other words TAU], would my method probably win then?

Wampold looked at me and said, "Not just probably: I would expect it to do so. You need a manual providing an explanation you can give to the client that makes sense and that persuade them to do something that is good for him or her."

In an elaboration of his response, Wampold told me about present-centred therapy (PCT), a form of intervention that was originally created as a control treatment for cognitive behavioural therapies for post-traumatic stress disorder (PTSD). The researchers in this instance needed a treatment that bore no resemblance to the cognitive behavioural methods under study, and so they put forward the idea of PCT. PCT had no plausible basis and no treatment manual; the therapists did not believe it was a proper treatment form. However, in order to ensure a satisfactory control treatment in a RCT study, the researchers added therapeutic ingredients based on psychological principles, produced a manual, and taught therapists how to carry out the treatment in a credible fashion. PCT was intended to represent the antithesis of cognitive behavioural approaches defined as trauma-focused.

PCT focuses primarily on present functioning, even though it doesn't explicitly state that one cannot speak about former traumas. The therapist gives the client information on how trauma can affect people's functioning and teaches strategies for solving associated problems. In trauma-focused therapies, on the other hand, it is important that the client confront the trauma by reviewing the traumatic event itself, and the thoughts and feelings connected to it. It is today generally accepted that trauma-focused treatment is the best form for treating PTSD. However, as Wampold says, perhaps one should look at the research one more time. There are currently three RCT studies that compare PCT with established, evidence-based treatments. These studies found that PCT is equally or more effective than the treatments with which it was compared. In two of the studies, there was also a significantly lower dropout level with PCT.

For me it is not difficult to believe the results, because I have experienced this in daily clinical practice. I have had clients for whom trauma-focused interventions have been critical for their improvement, and I have had clients for whom the focus on solving problems here and now has been more helpful. Often, the right approach has been a combination of the two. The common element is that I listened to the client to determine what might fit the unique individual sitting in front of me.

Most of what we do in a therapy session is fundamentally common sense. In the age of evidence, common sense has acquired a low status and is considered somewhat unprofessional. A public health nurse I know told me they could no longer recommend prunes for children suffering from constipation. No research has been done on this, and there wasn't sufficient evidence in support of prunes. When she was a child, my own daughter ate a pear for breakfast every morning, which worked miracles for her digestion. We were advised to do this by a public health nurse. One would have to search far and wide for such advice these days. In fact, a large amount of traditional advice has served people well over the years, but now has essentially been removed from the list of helpful tips (state guidelines) because we have insufficient evidence.

Knowledge about culture

In recent decades a lot of time and resources have been invested in researching methods and findings about different disorders and ailments, which have often resulted in the development of a diagnosis. However, repeated empirical research studies have shown that on average it is not the specific factors of methods that are decisive and that psychological problems do not always fit neatly into specific categories. Many researchers have argued that this is because we have not made enough progress with the research and that with more research we will learn and know more. Eventually, we will establish what is specific and distinctive, which will tell us what we should do when we encounter a specific type of problem. After several decades of continual confirmation of the irrefutability of the dodo bird verdict and an increasingly critical view of the diagnosis system, we can certainly state that now it's enough. We need more research. But we need another type of research.

In the age of diagnoses and methods, knowledge about culture and context has faded into the background. It is too complicated to fit into the scientific model. It would have been so much simpler with a common set of problems and common methods that could be applied universally, but that's not how it works.

In the book *Crazy Like Us*, author Ethan Watters (2010) takes to task the globalization of the Western manner of understanding the psyche. He uses examples to demonstrate how the Western, particularly American, understanding of psychological ailments spreads to other parts of the world. This has led to a dramatic increase in the incidence of psychological disorders with American labels in many parts of the world. The Western understanding of these disorders and their corresponding treatment protocols has transformed into an international conception that is believed to have cross-cultural application. Although this attempt to help people suffering from psychological disorders may stem from good intentions, it has lacked reflection about the consequences of such an approach. The way a culture thinks about psychological problems, how it categorizes and prioritizes the symptoms and seeks to cure them, and the expectations for prognoses and results also have an impact on the disorders themselves.

Watters offers examples of how individual diagnoses have been exported to other cultures and subsequently acquired a different content and scope from what they had at the outset. The increase of anorexia in Hong Kong, the understanding of schizophrenia in Zanzibar, and the marketing of depression in Japan all came about because the disorders acquired their own distinctive character in these cultures. Then they were Americanized and ascribed new meaning, contents, and another understanding of treatment. They also increased in scope.

We have already seen the problems related to believing that some methods provide better treatment than others using trauma therapy above as an example. Watters demonstrates a deeper understanding through his example of how PTSD was exported to Sri Lanka when the tsunami flooded the island and how cultural specificity was largely ignored. When the catastrophe struck Sri Lanka at Christmas time in

2004, there were a number of Western health care workers in the country. One of these was Debra Wentz, head of a psychological health organization in the USA. During the days following the tsunami she worked against the clock to prepare the country for the psychological catastrophe the population was now facing. She informed the prime minister about the psychological damages known as PTSD and the anxiety and depression that would grow as a problem and last for generations. Through the media, she informed the population of the symptoms of PTSD, fitting them into three different categories: avoidance, numbness, and hyperactivity. She advised everyone to be on the lookout for pathological behaviour in both adults and children and that for PTSD there was a need for professional treatment. The need for psychological health assistance after the tsunami would be greater than the world had ever seen, but how would Sri Lanka be able to address this without a sophisticated psychological health scheme or professionally trained therapists? Wentz started creating a plan that would make it possible to send American trauma experts to Sri Lanka to train local therapists in how to detect and treat PTSD. She undoubtedly had a genuine desire to help a nation in need and sacrificed both her time and energy for the greater good. Her measures were motivated by assumptions about the fundamental nature of psychological trauma and about suitable treatments. She believed that the psychological reaction to trauma was the same all over the world.

Wentz wasn't the only one who sounded the alarm about the imminent psychological health catastrophe. Psychological health experts from all over the world could tell the media that millions of people in the near future would be afflicted with PTSD. What took place during the following months in Sri Lanka, Indonesia, India, and Thailand was very likely the largest international psychological intervention in history. Trauma therapists and researchers flooded into the region to give the population "modern" psychological health care. The idea that people from different cultures can have fundamentally different psychological reactions to traumatic events was difficult to comprehend.

Western trauma experts have viewed trauma as an individual problem, which must also be treated individually. Professionals were supposed to intervene at an early stage. Retelling the story of the trauma, along with the accompanying feelings and thoughts, was considered essential. These ideas were assumed to be universal. Out of all the trauma therapists who arrived in Sri Lanka in the weeks following the catastrophe, there were very few who had much understanding of the culture they were about to step into. Few of them understood the local language; they had little knowledge about religious denominations, grief and burial rituals, or the country's long and complicated civil war history. As one therapist stated, "If one is going to provide psychological health treatment that is the equivalent of putting a compress on a head injury, why does one then need to share the person's religious faith, traditions, or social structures?"

There were those who protested. The University of Colombo in Sri Lanka issued a statement, requesting that the legion of therapists and counsellors who arrived in the country not reduce the experiences of the bereaved to a matter of "psychological trauma". For the locals, the traumatic event would be interpreted in light of the society and culture in which it occurred. In turn, this would determine how the survivors sought help and the expectations they had for healing. Trauma reactions are not automatic psychological reactions in the brain of an individual but rather a part of a cultural communication. They have nuances and meanings that can be misinterpreted or overlooked if the observer does not have a deep understanding of the culture in which they occur. What was required before any international organization could offer meaningful assistance was an understanding of what the affected individuals tried to express in their time of need. Without this, it would be impossible to offer any meaningful form of care.

It is when I meet people from other cultures that I truly understand how different people are and how futile it is to place somebody in a category or define them according to a checklist. The philosopher Plato wrote, "Then anyone who leaves behind him a written manual, and likewise anyone who takes it over from him on the supposition that such writing will provide something reliable and permanent, must be exceedingly simple-minded." By categorizing people, we miss essential knowledge that we need to help them. We fail to obtain the context and culture.

"If we can't laugh at ourselves, we might as well just end it all," a Catholic woman, who was a foreigner living in Norway, once said to me. She had just suffered a great loss, but I laughed so loudly during our first session that they heard me in the next room. Her doctor was concerned about her grief reaction, and that was why she was sitting in my office. During the entirety of the first session, we spoke of her upbringing, how people reacted to different events in her culture, the relationship to grief, and how she and her Norwegian husband grieved in different ways. The entire conversation took place in her mother tongue, so she could express herself in her own way, with her unique, sardonic humour in what was the most difficult period of her life. If I had attempted to tick off her reactions on a checklist of symptoms, I would never have learned how to help her move forward in her life. If I had tried to impose a treatment process on her that was a bad fit, she probably would not have come back.

Cultural differences do not occur only between countries or continents. They also appear within local communities. In the municipality of Stange, a densely built-up urban area of Ottestad borders the city of Hamar. There are large farmsteads in the district of Romedal, small holdings in Vallset, and a theatre and music community in Tangen. I meet people from all these communities, and each has distinctive ways of understanding and solving life's difficulties. Therefore, I can't take it for granted that I know something about a person based on a description of symptoms, or disorder category. First, I must ask questions about and explore the person's life-world.

I learned about it on Twitter

We need broad understanding, knowledge that extends far beyond the scope of methods or categorized disorders. Unfortunately, acquiring knowledge can be a challenge. As a student, I could only use the Internet to do searches of journal databases where I could find information about various subjects in the form of research articles. Now I use mostly Google and social media. Through Facebook and Twitter, I receive updates on what is happening in the field and links to new research. These are often posted by trade unions, user organizations, other organizations within the field, or private individuals with expertise in psychology and therapy. Knowledge derived from journal articles is fine, and we need a lot of it, but there is so much more. Of course, there is good reason to be sceptical about a lot of the information on the Internet. We risk gaining only superficial knowledge by educating ourselves, limiting ourselves to fragments of online information that do not cover a topic in sufficient depth. In the book *Bad Science*, author and psychiatrist Ben Goldacre (2008) exposes questionable interpretations of research findings and the ways both the media and researchers disseminate research as they see fit. Knowing how to read research results critically is just as important as possessing subject expertise. This critical eye enables us to guide clients in sifting through information they find on the Internet and identify what is might actually be helpful to them.

Sigrun Tømmerås, whom we met in the first chapter, provided me with some important lessons about psychology and therapy. After hundreds of her newspaper articles had been published, two Swedish cyber friends encouraged her to start a blog. Tømmerås told me that she didn't understand how one could reach people with a blog, but they kept pushing her, so she decided to give it a try.

> In 2008, the number of active bloggers was far less than it is today. But there was a good blogger community, and I was well received. At that time, there weren't very many writing about mental health or writing from a critical perspective. But I was invited in from the cold, and with time, nominated for blog contests. It was a nice experience, almost like falling in love.

Tømmerås was awarded a prize for the promoting freedom of expression in mental health care after having blogged for nine months. Shortly thereafter, she started using Twitter.

> It was a big deal among bloggers then, and you felt a little out of it if you weren't on there. However, I don't know if I have the same credibility on Twitter as others, because I have a diagnosis. Once, there was a psychologist and journalist who wrote about scientologists and claims about psychiatry's ties with the pharmaceutical industry. When I remarked that this is actually true, the response I got was that there was an abundance of conspiracy theories about this. After I posted a link to a journal that confirmed my claim, there was no response.

Tømmerås often posts links to articles in journals and newspapers, reports, and other sources that address mental health. Subscribing to her blog (https://stomm-blog.blogspot.com/) or watching her Twitter account helps keep me up to date on recent developments in the field.

Tømmerås is critical about what she posts. As a trained librarian she knows what she is sharing.

> I have appointed myself to be a public educator; I am not a librarian for nothing. I subscribe to several newsletters and feeds. For several years, I have also subscribed to the Norwegian Psychological Association's journal, which was helpful in the aftermath of a horrendous therapy experience. After the treatment was terminated, I couldn't stand words such as psychology or psychologist. One time, I was at the university bookstore and just had to run out when I saw the shelves of psychology books. Then I submitted articles to the journal and started to subscribe in 2007 when they printed the third piece. At first, my heart would start pounding when I saw it in my mailbox, and I could barely manage to tear off the plastic wrapper. "Psychology stuff" was so ominous. Now I seldom read anything that produces this kind reaction.

We need many different kinds of knowledge to be good helpers. Many of us have a lot of expertise, but we need to use the entire range of our knowledge. We must remember that the most important thing is to acknowledge when we don't know something. This is hard work, but it's worth it.

Well-informed and wise

We can be well informed, and we can be wise. We become well informed by reading a lot, familiarizing ourselves with the most recent research and by practising new skills. We become wise only when we combine knowledge with experience and reflection. Most of us have a lot of knowledge and a lot of experience, but we can live an entire lifetime without this making us particularly wise. We become wise only when we reflect on the consequences of what we have done; did our actions produce the desired effect or not? If we keep repeating the same mistakes or continue doing something that is not helpful, we do not become wiser at all, but instead dumber. By learning from our mistakes and reflecting upon our experiences, we can hopefully become a bit wiser with age. Wise professionals are able to combine experiences with knowledge. In the next chapter we are going to learn about the first step on this path, specifically soliciting feedback.

3

FEEDBACK

Feedback is the breakfast of champions.

Ken Blanchard

Gard: This car has six gears, you know.

Birgit: Hmph! [changes gears]

Gard: I've been sitting here a long time without saying a word.

Birgit: I'm the driver, I know how to change gears.

Gard: You usually forget.

Birgit: We were driving uphill.

Gard: A mile back.

Birgit: I know when to change gears.

Gard: You usually forget.

Birgit: Hmph!
(A conversation while out for a drive)

Feedback is an important and everyday part of communication between human beings. We do it all the time. Still, it is hard to both give and take feedback. Positive feedback is what we need the most. It strengthens us as individuals and helps us develop good self-esteem. Positive feedback is crucial for healthy development in children and a vital element of any good working environment or friendship. On the other hand, feedback that is intended to improve one's performance by illustrating where we can be more effective (which we will call "negative" and/or "corrective" feedback) is more difficult. The aim of this kind of feedback is to correct us when we are going off track or to let us know how we might be better. In this book, I speak mostly about corrective feedback, not because I believe the positive kind is less important – quite the contrary. However, because correction is necessary for us to learn and excel at anything, negative feedback is wholly indispensable. Ultimately, the goal is to improve and not to feel bad about ourselves. As the psychology researcher Helene Nissen-Lie and her colleagues (2015) state, the therapist should "Love yourself as a person [and] doubt yourself as a therapist."

The most problematic aspect of negative or corrective feedback is that it tells us that we are somehow wrong, and this can be painful. In her book *Being Wrong*, journalist and author Kathryn Schulz (2010) demonstrates why it is so fundamentally difficult for human beings admit that we make mistakes, even though we do so all the time. While we experience being right as a normal state of affairs, being mistaken is something rare or unnatural. We often feel foolish and embarrassed. We lose confidence and would prefer just to forget about it. Still, we can learn a lot about ourselves by recognizing our own fallibility. Twelve hundred years before René Descartes wrote his famous words "I think, therefore I am," the theologian and philosopher Augustine of Hippo wrote *Fallor ergo sum*: "I am wrong, therefore I am". Being wrong is not just a part of being alive; it is proof that we are alive. By embracing our mistakes, we can benefit and learn from them. Schulz writes that all mistakes are demonstrations of optimism. We make mistakes because we believe in ourselves, even though we have not succeeded before. Making mistakes is about hope, because when we accept our mistakes, in the belief that we have learned something, our hope is that we will get it right the next time around.

One of the most important elements we need to achieve success and become better at something is feedback. Without feedback on what we do, it would be extremely difficult for us to improve ourselves. This chapter will discuss how to acquire systematic feedback in a therapeutic setting, which is an important tool for professional development and providing the best possible service.

The start of feedback research within psychotherapy

Michael Lambert spent the first years of his research career investigating treatment processes with negative outcomes. It wasn't until the 1980s that he became interested in how to prevent such negative processes. He had spent a lot of time determining what caused them but had made no attempt to prevent their occurrence. That was when he began to develop an interest in measuring treatment effect. It started when a large mental health service provider in the USA contacted him, wanting to hire him as a consultant. They wanted his help selecting outcome measures for all their clients, so they could start measuring results. At the time, there were few such outcome measures. In particular, the company wanted a way to identify when there was a risk of a negative outcome, which led to Lambert personally developing the outcome questionnaire (OQ45).

OQ45 is a self-reporting tool made up of 45 questions that can be answered at different points in the course of the treatment process (Gleave, Burlingame, Beecher, et al., 2017). The tool contains three subscales: symptom distress, interpersonal relationships, and social role, which combine to measure overall disorder distress. If a person experiences improvement, this will be evident on the OQ45. The first version of OQ was published in 1992 and proved effective for identifying clients in danger of a negative development during the course of therapy. The challenge was to get therapists to use it with all their clients in every session. Thus, Lambert and his group continued to develop OQ, shortened it, and developed software that provided therapists with timely and ongoing feedback on the client's therapeutic progress. Today Lambert is considered a pioneer in this field and has inspired many other researchers to take an interest in feedback. He and his research team at Brigham Young University in Utah are still working on further development of feedback tools with an eye to making them more precise and applicable in many different contexts.

My start as a psychologist – Hagen treatment centre

My first job as a recently certified psychologist was at the Hagen treatment centre. It was purely by coincidence that I ended up at this little mental health care institution for children in Veldre, Ringsaker, Norway. After I completed my education, my husband and I decided to move to Hamar, and I scoured the psychology journal in search of job vacancies in the region. This was right before the summer holiday, and in the June edition of the journal there was only one position for a psychologist in the field of children's mental health advertised in the area – at Hagen. I applied and was called in for an interview on a gorgeous summer day in July 2004.

After driving back and forth a bit up on the hillside, I finally found my way to Hagen, which had formerly been a farm. Tove Huggins, the director of the centre, came up the hill to the car park to meet me and we sat down together on a bench in the sunshine with a view over the entire property. In front of me were the old farmhouse, the barn, and a traditional Norwegian storehouse, which originally comprised the farm buildings. When the buildings were first put to use as an institution, a schoolhouse and office module had been added. She told me about the facility's history, and already I began to sense that this was a wholly special place.

After the first introduction we moved into the office module and sat in the meeting room to start the actual interview. Huggins asked me challenging questions, because it was clear she knew what qualities she wanted in those she hired at the centre. At one point she asked me: "Are you concerned about being clever?" I hadn't thought very much about that, but I answered that I was concerned about ensuring that the families I met experienced that what we did together actually helped them. I added that, if it wasn't helping, I would try to do things differently and better. She told me that at Hagen they used continual evaluations from the parents on how they experienced the treatment, and it was also expected that I would do the same. With fresh from my academic experience, I said that that sounded like an extremely sensible practice, in which I would gladly participate.

I got the job and worked at Hagen for four years. This was an important time in shaping the direction I chose as a psychologist and how I relate to the entire field of mental health care. I was deeply affected by the mindset that was already well established in practice at Hagen.

Feedback-Informed Treatment (FIT)

I hadn't been working there for many months before Huggins sent me to a training with Scott Miller. Much sought after as a lecturer who has written several books and articles, Miller is the founder of the International Center for Clinical Excellence, a coalition of researchers, clinicians, and instructors who are interested in what promotes performance excellence within the mental health care field. At an early stage, he developed an interest in the use of feedback tools. During the years I was working at Hagen, I attended several courses and conferences with Miller and his colleagues, in both Norway and the USA. I have had extensive conversations with him about the use of feedback tools and the research behind them.

I asked Miller if he would be interested in a conversation in connection with this book and he agreed. He has often lectured in Norway, and on this occasion I met him at a cosy inn located in the Finnskog region, where he had come to give a training. Miller started by telling me about his own beginnings as a young psychologist. He wanted what every recent psychology graduate wants: to find out how to carry out therapy in the best possible manner. He observed that many of the other students seemed more self-confident about how they should talk with people, and everything seemed very clear and evident for them. That was not the case for Miller. He wanted to offer help that was effective, but asked himself questions all the time about how he could accomplish this.

"When one asks this question within psychotherapy, the field does not have a shortage of answers," Miller said:

it has a wealth of answers. Confront dysfunctional mindsets, analyse feelings, think about the childhood, move the finger back and forth, dots on somebody's face, group therapy, take medication – for me this was very confusing. Those espousing each and every one of these approaches professed great faith in their procedures, something which for me went against all logic. These people could observe the same therapeutic interaction and describe it in completely different ways. How could all of this be right? I was really confused.

In the period that followed, Miller spoke with almost all the therapists he knew and attended as many courses as he could up until the time he met Insoo Kim Berg and her team. She was interested in solution-oriented therapy, and over a two-year period Miller learned this method inside and out. He watched hour after hour of therapy sessions and eventually practised the method with facility and felt more secure. Then the team had some outside researchers come and study the effect of the therapy more closely. The results showed that solution-oriented therapy was not more effective than any other approach, which triggered a crisis of faith for Miller.

I had finally mastered being a therapist, I was not anxious about being in the same room with a client, and then it turned out that what I did was no better than anything else. So in a way I was back where I'd started. It wasn't that the knowledge about solution-oriented therapy didn't help people, it did. But it wasn't unique and I wanted to find out what really was helpful.

Miller was at a crossroads. He had become a confident, solution-oriented therapist with great belief in his method, but then it turned out that the method wasn't any better than other methods. This bothered him. Countless models and methods had been developed in the field, all of which claimed to be effective. There is something wrong with this, Miller thought: they can't all be effective and explain causes in so many different ways. That was when he began looking at the common factors. As a student, Miller had studied under Michael Lambert at university, but, when Lambert spoke about common factors at that time, Miller didn't think it sounded particularly exciting. He explained:

What was exciting was diving into the unconscious mind of a person or learning neurobiology. These approaches had more depth and

> roots. Lambert mixed so many things together – salt, pepper, flour, the basic ingredients of an approach, but it provided an understanding of why there could be so many explanations for the different methods, while the results achieved were essentially the same.

For a long time, Miller was interested in the common factors and believed this constituted an adequate explanation, but eventually he realized it was not enough:

> The minute you start talking about common factors over time, then the therapists want to learn how they can make use of them. And then you have a philosophical problem, because as soon as you say: "Here's the way to apply the common factors," you have proposed a new method. And so you are back to specific methods. This led me to measurements, because what one wants to know is whether what one is doing actually works.

In the course of the years that followed, Miller and his colleagues developed a method known as the *Partners for Change Outcome Management System* (PCOMS), and subsequently *Feedback-Informed Treatment* (FIT), described below. On its own, PCOMS (a recognized evidence-based practice) is comprised of two scales that provide therapists with client feedback about whether they are experiencing improvement and how they experience the alliance with the therapist. These are the Outcome Rating Scale (ORS) (Miller, Duncan, Brown, Sparks, & Claud, 2003), which measures changes in overall well-being, and the Session Rating Scale (SRS), which measures the client's assessment of the therapeutic alliance. Several studies have established that the scales are reliable, valid, and user-friendly. They were initially developed for adults, with later scales produced for children: the Child Outcome Rating Scale (CORS) and the Child Session Rating Scale (CSRS). What is unique about these tools is that they give the client an opportunity to influence the collaboration and play a key role when it comes to deciding treatment design.

The ORS is a visual analogue scale on which the client can offer feedback in four different areas regarding how he or she is feeling. Each area has a 10-centimetre line, and the client marks a cross or a dash on the line. The closer to the right the client places the mark, the better the client feels he or she is doing, and the worse they are feeling, the closer to the left they place the mark.

The therapist then places a ruler on the lines and calculates a score. The highest possible score is 40. The clinical cut-off score on ORS is 25 for adult clients (32 for children and 28 for adolescents). That means that scores over 25 for generally indicate that a person is not experiencing distress at the same level as those who typically seek mental health services. Those who score below 25 are often seeking help in order to feel better. Some of those who seek help may score above 25, but often have a specific problem they wish to address. If the help they receive is successful, the ORS scores will go up. To monitor this, the scores are plotted on a graph. The therapist then receives feedback on whether the ORS score is within the range of the "expected response to therapy". These graphs resemble and have a similar function as the growth curves for weight, height, and head circumference that are used to measure a child's development compared to the average in the population. To access such information you can use a web-based program such as FIT-Outcomes (www.fit-outomes.com).

The SRS works in the same way as ORS, except in this case the therapist wants feedback on how the client experiences their collaboration. This scale is thus completed at the end of the session. SRS asks the client for feedback in four areas. The client provides input about whether they felt heard, understood, and respected; whether we worked on what they wanted to work on; if the approach suited them; if the session as a whole was good; and if something was missing. By filling out this scale, the client gains an opportunity to say something about how he or she experienced the meeting with the therapist without having to express it verbally.

Through this feedback we gain insight into whether what we are doing is actually working for our clients. It is important to respond to the client's feedback clearly. When using the SRS, the client must see that what he or she reports is taken seriously. This does not necessarily mean that the therapist will do everything the client asks, but that we will take their wishes under advisement and discuss them with the client. Often clients have a lot to teach therapists about how we can help them, and this is a particularly good way to see into their inner world of ideas. For the use of ORS and SRS to function well, therapists must be open to negative feedback and adapt accordingly. It is vital to establish a feedback culture where clients recognize that their opinions and evaluations are just as significant as the therapists'. The therapist's flexibility can be decisive to reaching solid alliance. I have also noticed these scales do something to my own attitude. The method causes me to take my clients seriously, and I am constantly impressed by what they have to contribute and how much my efforts improve.

As noted above, PCOMS has been studied in many parts of the world, with very encouraging results. It has been listed as an evidence-based treatment by the National Registry of Evidence-Based Programs and Practices in the United States. However, Miller and his colleagues were concerned that PCOMS did not, on its own, provide clear pathways for practitioners to improve. In order for clinicians to become more effective at their work, they must also engage in a course of deliberate practice, described in Chapter 4. When the measures that made up PCOMS were combined with deliberate practice, this became known as *Feedback-Informed Treatment* (FIT; Prescott, Maeschalck, & Miller, 2017).

Feedback scepticism

In the spring of 2012, I gave a lecture on the client's perspective of treatment for a group of leaders from the regional hospital trust, Helse Sør-Øst. In the talk, I addressed the importance of getting feedback from the clients and allowing it to guide the development of therapeutic services. The majority of those attending were interested and offered engaged and curious questions and comments. However, one woman was sceptical. In the course of this one hour, she asked all the critical questions I had often heard at the beginning of my career as a lecturer, but less frequently in recent years. This prompted me to look back on the time that had passed and the development that had occurred since then.

One of my first lectures was about the specialized studies programme at the Regional Center for Child and Adolescent Mental Health, Eastern and Southern Norway (RBUP) in 2006. Participants were predominantly therapists from the specialist health care services: child welfare educators, social workers, psychologists, and doctors. At that time, there were some enthusiastic audience members, but the sceptical voices were more evident. The most common objection was that the clients' mental states are so poor that their feedback could not be trusted. How could we know whether what they checked off on the feedback scales was true? Perhaps their answers were intended to placate us? Or they were so sick that they could not judge for themselves how they were feeling? Another objection was that it can take a very long time for somebody to get better, and improvement at the beginning of the process does not represent a real change. That would not happen until later, after many hours of therapy. Yes, many people in fact claimed that some clients must become much worse before they can get better and what use is an ORS graph then? Some clients were also in such a bad state that they couldn't get better, so the objective was simply to keep them stable. In such cases, we couldn't subject them to the ordeal of assessing how they were actually feeling. Some thought that such scales were destructive for the alliance and didn't want the interference they represented. Others maintained that it was not possible to measure whether somebody experiences a change in their life, and questioned the validity of the scales. These types of questions have diminished over the years, but they still pop up now and then. Some of the answers can be found in the research. For example, there is no research stating that to feel better one must first feel worse. For the most part, these questions are about a perspective on humanity and an attitude that maintains a distinction between us (professionals) and them (the clients) in the mental health field. The questions will be answered indirectly here as you read this book and by the time you have reached the end I hope you I will have assuaged some of your concerns.

Feedback research

"However beautiful the strategy, you should occasionally look at the results." Lambert uses this quote, often attributed to Winston Churchill, to open his chapter in the book *The Heart and Soul of Change* (Lambert, 2010). In the chapter, titled "Yes, it is time for clinicians to routinely monitor treatment outcome", Lambert addresses the feedback research within the field of psychotherapy up to the present day. Lambert and his research group had performed five large randomized controlled trials. In all the studies, the clients were randomly divided into two groups: for the first, the therapists received feedback, and in the second the therapists received none. To control for the therapist effect, the same therapists were used in both groups, and they applied a broad variety of treatment approaches. Each trial required approximately one year of data acquired from session-by-session collection of feedback and involved a total of more than 4,000 clients. The instrument used to measure improvement was the Outcome Questionnaire OQ45 (Lambert, Morton, Hatfield, et al., 2004). All the clients filled this out at every session and the individual results were compared with a normative data baseline (the expected treatment outcome). Those who did not experience the expected improvement were highlighted as not on track. The therapists who received feedback in this case were made aware of these clients by looking at graphs with colour-coded messages when the clients did not experience improvement. There was some variation in the five studies. Two gave both the therapist and the client feedback; two others looked at the effect of providing the therapist with feedback on the client's perception of the therapeutic alliance, which also included proposals for interventions (known as clinical support tools).

The results of the five trials were unambiguous. Giving the therapists feedback improved the results of clients at risk for negative outcomes. Providing further feedback on the alliance increased this effect and doubled the number of clients who experienced an improvement. The data also showed that when the therapists received feedback there was a decrease in the number of clients who terminated treatment with a negative development (from 20% to 13–15%). This was further reduced with feedback on the alliance along with proposals for solutions (at which point it dropped to 8%). In addition to having an impact on the results, feedback showed an influence on the length of treatment. The clients who did not experience any improvement remained in therapy longer than those in the control group. In other words, feedback prevented clients from dropping out before they experienced any improvement, allowing therapists to continue collaborating with clients and find solutions that worked for each individual. Clients identified as being on the right track had fewer sessions than those in the control group. This demonstrates that feedback helps the therapists give the right amount of treatment to achieve a positive outcome.

In recent years, RCT studies have explored use of ORS and SRS. Reese and his colleagues (Reese, Norsworthy, & Rowlands, 2009) did a study at an American university clinic, independent of the group that developed the client and performance-based practice that has evolved into Feedback-Informed Treatment (FIT). The results showed the feedback group achieved significantly greater change than the treatment-as-usual group and required fewer sessions. Morten Anker is a Norwegian psychologist affiliated with the child and family protection services in Norway. In 2009, together with his colleagues, he carried out the "Norway Couples Project", one of the largest studies on couples therapy in the world Anker, Duncan, and Sparks (2009). This research looked at the effect of giving both client and therapist systematic feedback on the client's assessment of progress in treatment and the alliance in couples therapy. The results showed that by the end of treatment couples in the feedback group experienced significantly greater improvement than those in the treatment-as-usual group. They achieved a clinically significant change that was almost four times greater and better outcomes six months after the termination of treatment. The feedback group also had significantly fewer cases of separation and divorce. There was almost 50% lower likelihood of couples in the feedback group going their separate ways six months later.

Resistance to feedback

The greatest obstacle to collecting client feedback is resistance on the part of the therapists. A number of studies have shown that most clients find it useful, and that it helps them focus on their own change process (Anker, Sparks, Duncan, Owen, & Stapnes, 2011; Sundet & Johansen, 2012). However, the objections on the part of therapists are many, which brings me back to the critical questions I received when giving a lecture. Can we trust the clients' feedback? I once had a few counselling sessions with a woman who was going through a difficult period in her life. When she filled out the ORS, she placed her marks quite far to the right, so she received a total score of 26. When she started telling me how she was feeling, it seemed to coincide poorly with how she had placed the marks. Based on what she told me, I would have expected her to place them much lower. I commented on this, which caused her to burst out rather spontaneously, "You know, one always lies a little bit on these kinds of forms." We both laughed a bit, and I explored this further. She said that she wanted to appear better than she was, and thought it was difficult to be completely honest, both with herself and with me. I asked her if she would consider marking her scores again now that we had reflected on this, and she gave them a significantly lower placement. At the end of the session she was supposed to fill out SRS. I said with a measure of levity in my voice that she now had to promise me that she'd be excruciatingly honest, so I would receive feedback on how we could collaborate in the best possible manner. She ended up giving the alliance a score that was quite low! This time she offered concrete opinions on what we had talked about that did or did not suit her, and we talked about how we could adjust the treatment in the next session to make it more meaningful for her.

The use of feedback tools in therapy is not an X-ray of the truth. It is a measure of what the client wants to communicate to us. How we relate to the feedback determines whether the scales are helpful, not simply the scales themselves. The vital element is that we are open, curious, and interested to hear what clients have to say, and make the necessary adjustments that will enable them to be as sincere as possible in their dialogue with us. Research tells us that these feedback tools are a more precise rendering of the clients' view of both improvement and the alliance than relying on the therapist's clinical judgement alone (more about this in Chapter 5).

Not long after I started working at Hagen, I became a member of the FIT network's working committee at BUP. We organized theme days, held practice seminars, and worked to promote the use of feedback tools in therapy by more mental health care professionals. In 2007 the book *Klienten – den glemte terapeut* ("The Client – the forgotten therapist") was published, on the initiative of the working committee (Ulvestad, Henriksen, Tuseth, & Fjeldstad, 2007). However, the efforts to generate interest in this subject felt irksome at times. Within the specialist health care services there was a lot of scepticism and reluctance; professionals felt they didn't need this type of information from their clients. They were focused on completely different things. Diagnoses had to be made, evaluations and reviews had to be completed, and plans had to be written – all tasks required by central regulatory bodies. The use of feedback tools was not a requirement and therefore not made a priority. There were moments when we had to recognize that feedback in therapy had not gained the level of investment that we'd envisioned, and we wondered if it ever would.

Then the tide began to turn. Gradually, as the RCT studies on the advantages of feedback were published, this type of tool was also recognized by professionals and regularly mentioned in guidelines and reports on good practice. At the same time, a change occurred within the Norwegian public health institution Helse-Norge. With increasing investment in low-threshold local services, more services were now provided closer to where people live. In local practices, the priority requirements had been changed, giving professionals more freedom, together with the clients, to design the services according to their needs. Feedback tools became a popular way of assuring the quality of services and increasing their efficiency.

In November 2012, Arild Bjørndal, the director of RBUP, invited us to a meeting. He had taken an interest in FIT (the method for incorporating client data into treatment) and was impressed with the research into the use of these types of scales. RBUP offers regular training in this treatment approach. He and others felt there was a need for research that could provide information about what happened in agencies where this approach had been implemented. On this occasion, researchers, instructors and directors at the workplaces where FIT is to be implemented are invited to discuss how this can be done.

I arrived bit early to the meeting and took the elevator up to the fourth floor of RBUP's premises in Nydalen in Oslo. When I entered the meeting room, only Morten Anker (who did the feedback study on couples therapy) had arrived before me, and we exchanged a few words about his ongoing projects. Shortly afterward, we were joined by Rolf Sundet, who also did his PhD based on FIT. He told us that five articles would be published internationally as a result of his work. Eventually more people arrived. The research department of RBUP was represented along with other external researchers, instructors like me, and representatives from a number of practices that had requested training in this approach. Everyone was enthusiastic and inspired. As the discussions unfolded around the table, it struck me how the attitude towards allowing the clients to tell us what they think about the help they receive had changed. This had become important, the hallmark of service. Any remaining scepticism was more about whether as professionals we were able to do this effectively, not about whether we could trust what the clients say. On the way out of the meeting I fall into conversation with a young psychologist, recently hired in a nearby municipality, who wanted to implement FIT. I told her how good it was to see optimism about this way of working. "Hasn't it always been like this?" she asks. "No, far from it," I answered.

User surveys function poorly as feedback

Linda Merethe Nordholm is a member of Mental Helse (the Norwegian national health, user, and interest organization) and a user representative. A few years ago, she was affiliated with the local child and adolescent mental health care outpatient clinic, where she assisted in their work of giving families an active role in designing their treatment programmes. The outpatient clinic is part of a larger health care enterprise, where all departments are required to carry out user surveys on a regular basis to evaluate the quality of the services. User surveys are a type of client satisfaction survey, which users of the service fill out anonymously after they have completed their treatment. The results from such user surveys are used to form the basis for improvement of the quality and efficiency of the services. The user surveys address, among other things, the availability of the services, information provided in advance and during the treatment process, how clients experience being met, follow-up after termination, the possibilities for influencing the treatment programme, and evaluation of own mental health. When Linda was hired by the outpatient clinic as a user representative, one of her duties was to look at how they could make better use of these user surveys. She did a thorough job, reviewing many of the responses and making suggestions for how the forms could be improved. Once, Linda told me about the response from one particular client. The response was anonymous, as user surveys often are, and was left in a mailbox in the waiting room. Linda described a young girl who had written at length about how she experienced the service. She hadn't merely checked off the correct boxes. She had written in the margins, at the top of the page, at the bottom of the page and essentially everywhere there was space available to express her views. This was a girl with a lot on her mind. Finally, Linda said, "Imagine how wonderful it would have been if this girl's therapist could have received this feedback!" Unfortunately, the therapist cannot, because the girl is anonymous and nobody knows who her therapist is.

One of the fundamental problems with most user surveys is that they have no real consequences for the individual therapist. They offer therapists no direct input on the work they are doing and therefore no opportunity to improve their relationship with the client giving feedback. The department as a whole will perhaps receive some feedback, but as a rule this will be so vague or general in nature that it will be difficult to make any practical changes. Individual responses communicating negative feedback cannot be understood as meaning that all the therapists should change. As long as one doesn't know which therapists have triggered a negative response, it is difficult to do anything. The clients also answer predesigned questionnaires defined by the health care personnel. It is conceivable that the client may want to communicate something else entirely about the treatment, like the girl who wrote in every available space on the form. What she wrote in the margins was not included in the numerical results of the survey.

Such user surveys tend to produce flattering results. In the health care services where they are used, it would seem as a general rule that a large majority of clients are satisfied with the services provided. This often corresponds poorly with the reality experienced by patient representatives, user organizations or other authorities that are approached by dissatisfied users. There is often a low response rate on user surveys. Those who are offered the chance to contribute to the survey are only the clients who have completed their treatment, while those who might have dropped out along the way have few opportunities for offering feedback. Some research has been done on the problems surrounding user surveys, which have generally addressed methodological questions. Regardless, the feedback from such surveys will be far too vague and unspecific for it to be useful in implementing actual changes.

When I speak about feedback from the clients, I am consequently not speaking about generic user surveys. In most cases, the resources required to conduct such surveys significantly outweigh the benefits derived from them.

Other forms of feedback

In psychotherapy, research on feedback considers whether or not the individual client experiences improvement. However, when a treatment provider is interested in using feedback to improve the quality of their service and its development, eventually they will seek out other types of feedback. We can become proficient therapists and work well with individual clients, but what is the mental health condition of the society in general? Has it improved, or is it almost the same? However proficient we may be with an individual client, we must always ask ourselves if this improves the field as a whole.

The first thing we can look at is whether the treatment "sticks" and any change that occurs in the clients is maintained. Return to therapy is one type of feedback that can demonstrate whether or not what we are doing is adequate. The number of returns to therapy is the first thing we look at, but the number offers little to identify where or what improvements are needed. It is not any more helpful than simply administrating ORS and SRS. What is important is how we receive this feedback and what we do with it. Returning to therapy is not necessarily a bad thing. While a client may experience improvement in one area, life may produce a renewed need for help. Likewise, just because you have been to see your family doctor once, it doesn't mean you will never need to go again. However, some of the returns to therapy may be due to the fact that the help the client received the first time around did not meet their needs. In such cases, it may be necessary to consider what these enquiries entail. Did the clients have an experience of learning to master their problems on their own, or did they become dependent upon the therapist, so that in the long term there was no sustainable improvement? Is the treatment provider essentially not prepared to address the issue at hand? In order to make effective use of feedback, it must be analysed and reflected upon. After that point, it can help the treatment provider to develop and move forward.

Dropping out is another type of feedback that tells us something about the quality of the work we are doing. Just as with returns to therapy, we must explore, analyse, and reflect upon what the cause can be for our missing something. It may then be wise to distinguish between those who drop out after having experienced improvement and those who drop out without having made significant progress. These two groups can have quite different reasons for terminating their treatment without this having been agreed upon first. The reasons why clients drop out can differ from one practice to the next. A good alliance between the client and the therapist can prevent dropout; that is also one of the reasons why use of the SRS is important. However, there will always be something that is missed, and finding out more about what we've missed can give us new opportunities to improve our services.

We can do a lot of reformation work to ensure that those who come to us for help experience improvement that they can maintain over time. What would really be interesting, however, would be to make a difference at a societal level. Have we had an impact on public health in the local community where the service is being provided? This type of feedback can track the number of people with a diagnosis, the number of people who take medication for mental health ailments, how many adolescents drop out of high school, how many people are on sick leave or receive disability insurance due to mental health ailments, messages of concern to the child welfare services, and the number of suicides. If we do not succeed in keeping these overriding issues in our minds, true advances will be difficult. The trend in society shows an escalating number of inquiries to both the mental health and child welfare services. One explanation has often posited that there is less associated stigma and more cases are thereby discovered, but if we succeed within our field, these inquiries should ultimately decrease. If we succeed in our work, including understanding how to work preventively, we should eventually see a tendency towards fewer serious mental health ailments. If the increase continues, we must acknowledge that we are doing something wrong. The increase in mental health disorders in and of itself is a form of feedback on how we are working and what should be changed. However, changes at this level are not something a single treatment provider can take responsibility for, but must instead be a joint endeavour spanning services and meeting places in society at large (Friedman, 2009).

Feedback for the future

In my conversation with Michael Lambert, whom I introduced in Chapter 1, we talked about his hopes for the future. He said he is optimistic about the research on feedback and continues exploring how to put feedback to better use and how clients function outside of therapy session. By gaining more feedback on this, we expand our focus to include interventions that are helpful in a larger social context, not solely within the walls of a therapy room.

We must continue to develop the field of feedback in the future and encourage interest in it on the part of the research communities. The qualitative measure of services should consider whether they contribute to improvement for the individual and better public health overall. How one uses one treatment method or the other is not a quality objective in and of itself. Different methods can make an important contribution to improvement. However, while we can't know whether one is better than the other, we should focus on the outcome of the help, not the merely mechanics of its application. Treatment methods will evolve and maintain a high level of quality when we become more interested in feedback on the outcome. That is inevitable.

Acquiring feedback is the first step towards making necessary improvements, but, if we stop there, not much will happen. This is simply where the work begins. Feedback has no real value by itself. It is how we respond to it that makes better therapy and improved outcomes. Improvement will come when we analyse and reflect upon the feedback we receive, and act upon it in the next round.

4

AFTER FEEDBACK COMES PRACTICE

Deliberate practice isn't what most of us do when we're "practicing".
Geoff Colvin

The story of WAP

The history of the mobile telephone is quite brief. The first official mobile telephone was purportedly used in Sweden by the police in 1946. But there wasn't anything especially mobile about it and it resembled more a two-way radio. Nor was it especially practical, because it used up the entire car battery in six phone calls. Throughout the course of the 1960s and 1970s, the technology continued to evolve through testing the mobile network. The design of the telephone itself was altered. It was still large, heavy, and so expensive that it was beyond the means of most people. It was not until the mid-1990s that the price and size of mobile phones made them practical for popular use. From then on, the design, contents and usage areas developed at a rapid pace up to the smartphone, which is virtually *de rigueur* today.

The mobile telephone industry is a user-controlled industry. What the manufacturers did not believe would catch on, such as text messages, has done just that. Meanwhile, features like WAP, which they believed would catch on quickly, did not. WAP (Wireless Application Protocol) was introduced at the end of the 1990s to give mobile phone users access to the Internet and email through mobile phones. The suppliers saw that the Internet had become a success and thought that Internet access on mobile phones would be equally successful. The problem was that they took the mobile telephone of that time and tried to make it access contents for which it was really not suited. By using WAP, Internet access on the mobile phone was possible, but only in text format, far removed from the Internet experience available on a computer. Tech companies worked hard to get people to use WAP and turn this into a commercial success, but the users didn't want it. They abandoned WAP, and the developers were forced to change their products. Public preference gravitated toward phones with a new kind of interface, which paved the way for the first smartphones on the market. End users got the contents they wanted in the format they wanted, and the entire industry took a huge leap forward as a result of changes prompted by user feedback. This is contrary to how so many psychotherapy methods are developed, in which new models and techniques emerge based on symptom reduction, but not necessarily client well-being or accessibility.

This chapter introduces the concept of *deliberate practice*, which has proven to bring about actual improvement in therapist performance. An important element of deliberate practice is feedback, as described in the last chapter. Now we will look first at what happens when we don't listen to feedback, then move on to learn how we can use feedback to achieve progress. Deliberate practice involves an approach or training exercise, coupled with coaching, with a clear intent toward advancement, improvement, or growth.

We don't listen to feedback from those suffering from mental health problems

Although the interest in using feedback tools within mental health care services is on the rise, there is not as much attention to listening to the feedback we receive from users. This persists in spite of the fact that several generations of clients have protested loudly about the nature of their encounters with health services. Inger Beate Larsen and Anders Johan W. Andersen at the University of Agder did a study in which they read and analysed 12 autobiographies written by patients from Norway, Sweden, and Denmark who had been involved with the mental health care system (Andersen & Larsen, 2012; Larsen & Andersen, 2011a, 2011b). The oldest book is from 1918 and the most recent from 2008. By studying these books published in different countries and different time periods, the researchers learned much about who these people are (or were), their experiences with mental health problems, and how they viewed the treatment they received.

Because the various autobiographies span a period of almost 100 years, one would think that the study would describe how psychiatry has changed over time. Psychiatry as a profession would probably also maintain that it has undergone radical changes during this period in terms of the mentality, treatment programmes, and understanding of mental health disorders. In the beginning of the 20th century, large asylum institutions prevailed. Three of the biographies are from this period. In the middle of the last century, antipsychotic medications were viewed as groundbreaking within psychiatry. Four of the books are from this time period. From mid-1980s up to today, the field of psychiatry has emphasized the proximity of services to the home and user cooperation. Four of the autobiographies are from this period.

Comparison of these autobiographies shows far more similarities than differences in the way the individual patients experienced their encounters with psychiatry. The researchers noted this as a clear contradiction with the perception of psychiatric history research as focused on change and progress.

The most pronounced feature of the books was the significance of being a whole person, independent of individual psychiatric diagnoses. Clients felt that being cared for and feeling respect were necessary.

They saw it as a matter of love, honesty, and willingness to cooperate. The surroundings were important, too. A home-like atmosphere where the individual could feel welcome and at home contributed to a far more positive treatment experience. This was something the authors of the autobiographies highlighted again and again. In terms of critique, the medication they were subjected to is the most frequently recurring theme, ranging from sedatives in the asylums in the first part of the 20th century and neuroleptics from the 1950s until today. Even the chemical intervention in its own right, which medical treatment for mental health ailments entails, was experienced as painful, regardless of the type of medication in question. This is because the side effects were considerable, self-control was reduced, and others took over.

The authors describe sessions and types of help received from psychiatrists as having many common features independent of time and place. The researchers maintain this can mean that the health care system in Norway and Scandinavia has not adjusted its fundamental understanding in the course of the more than 90-year-long period the study addresses, despite substantial, comprehensive changes in psychiatric treatment during the same period. Clients' experiences and attempts to speak up about what they thought of the health care system was not taken into consideration as new services were developed.

Andersen and Larsen's findings are supported by Swedish sociologist Lena Steinholtz Ekecrantz in her PhD dissertation (Ekecrantz, 1995): "In spite of major changes within psychiatric care in the last decades as documented in public reports, the patients' experiences of the encounter with psychiatry remain the same in most respects". Ekecrantz investigated the period from the 1950s to the 1990s in Sweden and observed the gap between the official psychiatric language and the patients' own experiences with psychiatry actually widened toward the end of the period. Relatively speaking, the patients have thus been more oppressed the closer we get to the present day.

When we don't listen to feedback, little progress occurs

Serious mental health disorders have probably been around at least as long as human beings have. Still, there has been little consensus regarding what these conditions are about and how to address them. The field appears to have advanced during the past 50 years. Researchers claim to have discovered biological causes for mental health ailments. The pharmaceutical industry has developed a number of medications. And the number of therapeutic methods has exploded. With all this progress, one would think that the number of people on sick leave or living on disability due to mental health ailments would have decreased over the past 50 years, but this has not happened. Today, mental health disorders are the most expensive of all causes of disability, while mental health disorders are among the most common causes of sickness-related absenteeism in Norway. Assistant managing director at the Norwegian Institute of Public Health Arne Holte calculated that mental health disorders cost society between 60 and 70 billion Norwegian kroner annually in lost earnings, social security costs, and treatment expenses. Public authorities estimate that half of us will be afflicted by a mental health disorder at some point in our lives. How have mental health disorders become one of the most common afflictions in the Western world?

Author and journalist Robert Whitaker addresses this question in his book, *Anatomy of an Epidemic* (2010). He attempts to explain why the number of mentally ill individuals on disability has tripled in the course of the past 20 years. The book looks at depression, anxiety, bipolar disorders, ADHD, and schizophrenia. Whitaker discusses the latter disorder with great concern because it appears that we are less effective at treating schizophrenia than we used to be. The treatment of schizophrenia has undergone many changes in the past 100 years. New medications have been introduced, brutal care regimens phased out, and a number of milieu therapeutic and psychotherapeutic methods developed. With the advances in research and treatment protocols since the beginning of the last century, one would expect to find increasingly better outcomes. Unfortunately, this does not appear to be the case. Whitaker outlines a 1994 Harvard report, which found that the outcomes for schizophrenia patients in the USA had become worse over the previous two decades and were not any better than they had been a century prior, which engendered his interest in finding out how this could possible. Later in the book he explores two sets of findings from the World Health Organization that the course of schizophrenia is better in developing countries than in the Western world. Explanations for this have been connected to social policy and cultural values, but it is also noteworthy that only 16% of the patients in developing countries were taking antipsychotics. In the Western world medication is common practice.

Anxiety and depression, diagnoses that formerly did not usually take people out of working life for long, are now common causes of disability status, in spite of the fact that an increasing body of medications and psychotherapeutic methods are in use. Some will maintain that too few get help early enough. However, is the problem that the methods are faulty or not readily available, or should we re-evaluate our entire understanding of mental health disorders? We need to look closer at the paradigm supporting our understanding and treatment of mental health problems. The medical model for mental health treatment has been through both crisis and success, but remains today the underlying platform when our services are expanded and developed. This is not a coincidence (Duncan, Miller, & Sparks, 2004).

Whitaker (2010) writes that great optimism reigned within psychiatry in the 1950s. New medications were developed, and researchers claimed to have succeeded in proving that a chemical imbalance in the brain is the cause of mental health problems. Two decades later, however, psychiatry had to acknowledge that it found itself in a deep crisis and had serious cause to fear for its own survival. Its first problem was that the medical explanation of mental health issues had a legitimacy problem. This was first articulated by psychiatrist Thomas Szasz in 1961. In his book, *The Myth of Mental Illness*, Szasz (1974) makes the argument that mental health problems are not medical in nature, but instead labels for people struggling with "life problems" or who behave in socially unacceptable ways. Several researchers followed suit. Authors as diverse as Michel Foucault, R.D. Laing, David Cooper, and Ervin Goffman have also questioned the medical approach to understanding mental health problems. They proposed instead viewing mental health issues as normal reactions to an oppressive society. Today, authors such as Lucy Johnstone continue to highlight the challenges facing diagnostic systems (Johnstone, 2015).

The second problem was an increase in the competition for patients. The therapy industry took off in the 1960s and 1970s as thousands of psychologists and other counsellors began offering their services.

Eventually, there were more non-medical therapists than psychiatrists. At the same time, there was disagreement within the ranks of the psychiatrists. Although many leaned toward a more biological form of psychiatry with an emphasis on medication, the Freudians continued to dominate at many educational institutions. While they found some help in the medications, they were convinced that mental health problems were psychological in nature. The social psychiatrists were also focused on the patient's environment. With these three approaches in conflict, the field experienced an identity crisis. Psychiatry had to struggle to survive.

The new antipsychotic medications failed to fulfil their promise. Patients resisted taking them, a reality expressed in the film *One Flew over the Cuckoo's Nest*. The reputation of benzodiazepines, for example, grew worse and worse. These medications were intended to be prototypes for the psychopharmacological revolution, but, once cast in a negative light, their sales dropped dramatically in the course of the 1970s.

In 1977, the American Psychiatric Association (APA) carried out a comprehensive campaign for remedicalization of the profession. The APA stressed the significance of making correct diagnoses with a focus on mental health problems as organic illnesses. Starting in 1974, Robert Spitzer led the work of revising the American Psychiatric Association's Diagnostic and Statistical Manual of Mental Disorders (DSM). In 1952, the DSM was a modest diagnostic manual of 132 pages. A newer version (DSM III), launched in 1981, had 494 pages. Conditions that had previously been viewed as a part of life's vagaries were now covered by a diagnosis, with reduced criteria for identifying a bona fide condition. The weight of the tome has continued to increase with each new edition. Published in 2013, the fifth edition of DSM (American Psychiatric Association, 2013) contains more than 1,000 pages. There's an old saying that, if you can't explain it simply, you don't adequately understand it. Perhaps there is something to that idea.

I was born and raised in the late 1970s and therefore don't have the same historical experience as my older colleagues. Many times, I have heard about the liberal conditions of the 1970s, when therapists did as they pleased. This was always explained as being something very negative, as if everything that was done back then was out of control and much of the work was not particularly effective. That could be right, but, as I sit and write about the history of psychiatry, I wonder about whether the work done at that time was appreciably worse than what therapists are doing now. We want so very much to believe that we have advanced with all the new measures that are implemented in this field.

My conversation with Michael Lambert reflected on this. He said that he believes the reason for insufficient progress in the field is that we put too much weight on the medical model – in other words, the psychiatric understanding. People are not constructed in this way, and our attempts to fit them into such a model will not lead to any professional development. There are certainly a number of researchers who hold that the psychotherapy we provide today is better than the psychotherapy of 50 years ago, but Lambert disagrees. If one is very specific and has a narrow focus on what is being studied, it can perhaps appear this way. It may seem that we have become more effective within small areas, but the overall impact on people in a larger context has not changed over the years.

The time has come to learn from feedback

At the inn in the region of Finnskog mentioned in the last chapter, the conversation with Scott Miller continued. Together with his colleagues, and the help of his feedback scales, little by little he learned a lot about therapists' outcomes. Time after time, what emerged were the large differences between individual therapists. For a long time, Miller believed this to be coincidental, wondering whether therapists' work didn't vary for better or worse over time. As he studied these therapists, however, the differences in the data became so glaring that it was clear some therapists were consistently better or worse than others. The differences could not possibly be incidental. The problem was that it was not possible to isolate what made some therapists better than others. In the enormous amount of research attempting to determine what distinguished the best therapists from the others, the hypothesis was that they had to be doing more of what worked. Still, this wasn't a satisfactory explanation. It turned out to be extremely difficult to determine what it is that the best therapists do that differs from the practice of those who are mediocre.

For a long time, Miller and his colleagues got nowhere. They searched through the relevant literature for something that could explain why some therapists consistently achieved better outcomes than others. They brought in outside expertise to no avail, and the entire project was about to be shelved when Miller stumbled across the work of the Swedish psychologist K. Anders Ericsson. Ericsson is a professor of psychology at Florida State University and considered one of the world's leading researchers on expert performance. He was editor in chief of *The Cambridge Handbook of Expertise and Expert Performance* (Ericsson, Charness, Feltovich, & Hoffman, 2006), a book that has awakened the interest of people seeking to ascertain why some people excel in their fields. On one of his many flights home from Europe, by chance Miller came across an article by Geoff Colvin in *Fortune* magazine about Ericsson's findings. Miller told me enthusiastically,

> The article pointed out that there is in fact something that makes some people better at what they do than others. And some people become extremely good at what they do. Reading the article was like turning on a light bulb for me. I had finally found something meaningful in the search for what characterizes the really effective therapists.

Experience that helps you improve is not the type of experience you have the most of

I have a lot of experience driving a car. Raised in a village, I got my driving licence as soon as I turned 18. I have, no doubt, spent thousands of hours behind the wheel, but my husband thinks I drive irrationally and with poor concentration. And he is absolutely right. The point is that I don't make any effort to try and improve. I think about a lot of other things while I am driving, such as what I am planning to write about, a movie I just saw, or where to go on our next summer vacation. I drive on autopilot. There are many of us who carry out our jobs in this way. We do what we have to do without giving it much thought afterwards. That is why the amount of time spent at work has only a weak correlation with performance after the first two years (Ericsson et al., 2006, p. 691).

Experience without feedback gets you nowhere, but neither is feedback alone sufficient. In order for feedback to have an impact on learning, it must be integrated with reflection on the part of the recipient. We need to know where the problem is, and subsequently what we have to do in order to improve. Feedback must lead to changes in the way we do things. Then, we must receive feedback on how the new behaviour is functioning and reflect upon whether this has brought us closer to our goal. Essentially, it is a matter of the quality of practice and training. Ericsson calls this type of training *deliberate practice* and defines it as:

> individualized practice activities especially designed by a coach or teacher to improve specific aspects of individual performance through repetition and subsequent adjustment. To receive the maximum benefits from feedback, the individual must monitor his or her training with full concentration, something which is hard work and imposes limits on the duration of daily training.
>
> (Ericsson & Lehman, 1996, pp. 278–279)

We will explore in further depth the nature of this type of practice and its requirements, but let us first look at an example from the life of my daughter Lise.

Lise is our third child. Like most parents of young children, one of the first important milestones in our children's lives is when they learned to walk. With our first child, we practised a lot. We bent down and held both his tiny hands and supported him as he toddled about. With stooping shoulders, we walked back and forth across the living room floor, letting go to give him the feeling of walking by himself and catching him when he started to fall. It didn't take long before he was walking just fine all by himself at the age of one year. With Lise it was different. Her motor skill development was relatively similar to that of her older brother up to the age of one. By then she was also able to stand and liked cruising around while supporting herself on chairs and tables. She also had a wonder walker. As parents, on the other hand, we did not have a lot of time to walk around stooping our shoulders with her, now that there were two older children with needs to be met. We had also heard all the time that children learn to walk when they feel ready. Lise was born in May and, based on our experience with the two older children's walking careers, we assumed that she would be walking by the summer. But the summer arrived and Lise still couldn't walk without support. For sure she'll be walking by the time kindergarten starts in the autumn, we thought, and carried her around on our backs all summer long.

Kindergarten started and Lise still couldn't walk without support. Later in the autumn I was going to have a guidance session with my supervisor of many years, the neuropsychologist Bjørn Einar Bjørgo. Following such sessions, we often used to trade stories of experiences with our children, since he also had young ones. I told him about Lise's walking development and said that at the public health centre they were also starting to become a little concerned. Bjørn Einar's response left no room for doubt: put the wonder wagon in the attic, and start practising. She is not practising when she is walking around with it. She is just enjoying herself. Her brain receives no signals telling her that there is room for development here. On the contrary, her brain thinks that the way Lise is walking with her wagon is how she's supposed to walk. No, Bjørn Einar said, you must start training her. Hold her so she receives exactly enough encouragement to correct her balance. She must feel off balance and manage to recover her balance again. And you must do it long enough each time for the brain to establish connections with the new skill it is learning. And you must do this frequently enough that she develops. Twice a day at least, morning and evening.

With this new input, I went home to my husband and told him about the training programme. We had to make this a priority and I ignored feeble protests about whether this also meant Saturday and Sunday mornings. After four days of this kind of training, Lise was able to walk by herself.

A short time after the walking practice experience with Lise, I discovered an amusing study (Adolph, Shrout, & Vereijken, 2003), in which American and Norwegian researchers looked at what caused babies to develop differently when it was time for them to learn to walk. They found out that the key factor was not height, weight, age, brain development or any other congenital trait, but the amount of time the child spent on trying to walk – in short, walking practice. However, the eagerness to dedicate energy to this type of practice can differ among children.

The image of children who are learning to walk is a good image for how it really feels to improve. We toddle forward unsteadily, without knowing whether we will fall on our face or on our behind. There is a feeling of insecurity involved which many will attempt to avoid. But the longer we allow ourselves to remain in such a state of insecurity, and allow ourselves to fall down along the way, the more quickly we will master the new skill. It is only through this type of training that we will experience advancement. Ericsson's research gives us insight into some fields that have experienced great advancement, such as sports, music, and mathematics. We can learn something from them. The current best high school time for the marathon in the USA beats the gold medal winner at the Olympics in 1908 by more than 20 minutes. A double somersault in diving was virtually forbidden as late as in 1924, and is now an everyday exercise. Roger Bacon, a mathematician from the 14th century, wrote that a person needed 30–40 years of study to master mathematics as it was understood at that time. Today this type of math is learned at the high school level. When Tchaikovsky wrote his violin concerto in 1878, he asked the famous violinist Leopold Auer to perform it. Auer studied the score and said no: he claimed that it was impossible to play the piece. It is now played by young violinists who are studying to become musicians. Neither the brain nor the physiology of human beings has changed to such a degree that this can explain the development within these fields. Instead, human beings have learned to perform much better using the abilities they have and the bar within the respective fields has been raised dramatically.

Deliberate practice – training that works

Everyone knows what it means to practise, because we do it all the time. We think that, if we do something a lot, with time we will get better at doing it. For example, I am fond of playing the piano. Previously I took lessons with a piano teacher and reached a level where I can read music and play easy arrangements. When I am seated at the piano, I like to enjoy myself as I play, preferably playing straight through an entire song, so the melody emerges. I have to look at the sheet music because I don't know the score by heart and I make a number of mistakes as I play. When I have played a piece of music once, maybe I will play it one more time and then I think that I've improved. The first few times I do this, I might improve a little, but then my evolution stops. Once when I was playing I heard my husband chuckling in the background: "You make the same mistake every time. It has almost become a part of the song." If I really wanted to improve my playing, I should have practised in a completely different manner. I would have to focus on the sections where I make mistakes, and play these over and over again until I had them down pat. I would have to take in all the feedback I received by hearing what it was I was playing wrong and improve these sections by practising repeatedly. Then I would have to combine these sections with the rest of the arrangement to create a good flow. But I don't do this, because it's quite tedious.

Deliberate practice, as Ericsson has explained it, is a relatively specific means of bringing about improvement. It is not just about hard work or doing something many times (Ericsson, Krampe, & Tesch-Romer, 1993). Examples from sports and music can teach us a lot because they are domains with which everyone is familiar. Later on, I will explain how we can employ deliberate practice within the field of mental health.

When we are going to learn something new, we first want to try and understand what the new skill requires, then put ourselves into situations where we can try it out. We focus on mastering the new skill without making too many mistakes. As we gain more experience, we master the skill better; visible errors are diminished. Our performance seems to proceed more smoothly and we no longer need to concentrate as much on maintaining an acceptable level. After a limited period of experience, often less than 50 hours for most activities, we may have achieved a basic competence. We adapt to this level, and our performance becomes automatic, so we can perform the skill without much effort. At this automatic phase of learning, we reach a level that is stable, and there is little improvement thereafter. More experience will not lead to improved performance. This tends to be the case for driving a car, tennis playing, writing on a computer or playing chess. Daniel Kahneman, professor of psychology at Princeton University and winner of the Nobel Prize in economics, describes how our brain functions in situations that are especially mentally demanding. Attempting to solve mentally demanding tasks over a period of time is not particularly pleasurable, and we will therefore avoid it for as long as possible. Kahneman (2011) calls this "the law of least effort". We are not willing to push ourselves to achieve more than that which is strictly necessary.

Those who excel in their fields will continue improving with more experience as long as deliberate practice is involved. Deliberate practice is characterized by a number of elements. It is a matter of actions specially designed to improve performance, often with the help of a teacher.

Actions are repeated often, and the performer has ongoing access to feedback. It is mentally demanding and not much fun. Let us look at each element.

Identify what one needs to improve

The key to remember here is that this is a goal-oriented, thoroughly considered action. Usually, it must be done together with a coach, teacher or supervisor. This is important not solely because of the teacher's knowledge, but also his or her ability to see you in a way that you are unable to see yourself. Identifying the areas needing improvement is a demanding exercise. Noel Tichy, professor at the University of Michigan, illustrates this by drawing three circles, each one outside of the former. He calls the innermost circle "the comfort zone", the middle circle "the learning zone" and the outer circle "the panic zone". It is only by choosing activities located in "the learning zone" that one will achieve improved performance. We will never make progress in the comfort zone, because this entails activities we can already do easily, while activities in the panic zone are so difficult that we have no idea how to approach them. Identifying the learning zone is not easy. Compelling oneself to remain there as it gradually shifts, something that is even more difficult, is the primary and most important aspect of deliberate practice.

Repetition

The more frequently you repeat an action, the easier it becomes to get better at it. However, repeating an action many times, something most of us view as practice, will not necessarily cause you to improve. You also need feedback and reflection.

Feedback on the outcome must always be available

Practising without feedback is like playing golf and guessing where the golf ball lands, without checking to see if you are right. You can then hit the ball many times, but improvement will be virtually impossible, because you don't know what you need to change from one stroke to the next. For many activities, gaining feedback is a fairly simple matter, but when the results require interpretation it is crucial to have a qualified to provide feedback that will help ensure continued progress.

Deliberate practice is mentally demanding and involves reflection

First and foremost, deliberate practice requires a high level of discipline and concentration. When we have received feedback, we must reflect upon it to find alternative actions in order to bring about further improvement. This element of deliberate practice is yet another reason why so few of us undertake it. It is simply too demanding. We can only maintain such concentration for a limited and isolated amount of time. Those who perform best within their field only practise for approximately one hour without resting, and they prefer to practise in the morning, when they are rested. In most fields, four to five hours a day of deliberate practice appears to be the limit of what anybody can manage. Breaks between sessions is also common. If one doesn't limit the number of hours spent on this kind of concentrated training without getting enough rest between sessions, one can risk over-training or burn-out. Leopold Auer, the world famous violinist, is reported to have said, "Practice with your fingers and you will need the whole day. Practice with your thoughts and you will achieve just as much in an hour and a half."

Do what's required

Deliberate practice is not necessarily fun. In the early 1990s, a study was done at the Academy of Music in West Berlin to find out why some violinists were better than others. This academy was well known for educating extremely proficient musicians, many of whom went on to play for important symphony orchestras or to soloist careers. The professors were asked to point out the very best violinists, those with the potential for becoming international soloists. They were also to identify those who were very good, but not as good as those in the best group. The academy also had a department in which the admission requirements were less strict, with students who often became music teachers, and the researchers also recruited a group from this department. They now had three groups – good, better, and best.

The researchers then collected biographical data about the students. How old they were when they started playing, which teachers they'd had, the competitions they taken part in, and many other things. This data confirmed the evaluations of the music professors. The best violinists had had greater success in competitions than the better students, who in turn were more successful than those who were merely good. The students were then asked about how many times a week they'd practised every year since they started. They received a long list of activities, both music-related and non-music-related, and were asked how much time they had spent on each individual activity in a typical week. They were then supposed to rank the relevance of each activity in terms of making them better violinists, how tiring it was, and how fun it was. They were asked a number of other questions, as well, including how they had spent the day before, minute by minute. Then they were asked to keep daily journals for a week. Since journal reports are not always precise, the researchers double-checked them against other sources.

The results from all this data were straightforward and clear. In many areas, the three groups were the same. They started playing the violin at approximately the same age (eight years old) and decided to become musicians around the age of 15. Upon completing their studies, everyone had studied music for at least 10 years. What was most striking was that all three groups spent the same amount of time on music-related activities – lessons, practice, classes etc. – approximately 51 hours a week. The violinists were also reasonably sure about which type of activity was the most important in order to improve: solitary practice. Everyone knew this, but not everyone did it. There were great disparities in the amounts of time the different groups spent on solitary practice. The members of the two best groups practised alone an average of approximately 24 hours a week. The third group members practised alone nine hours a week. The groups also agreed that this was hard work and not particularly amusing, and that was the reason why only some of them did it. The importance of solitary study is clear in other fields as well. One of the reasons the best chess players can come up with so many alternative moves in such a short period of time is that they spend up to four hours a day on solitary study. They study and analyse previous games played by the best players in the world to find out how they can refine their own game.

Once familiar with this working method, one sees these principles applied everywhere performance excellence is found. In December 2012, Magnus Carlsen was ranked the best chess player of all time. In an interview on the Norwegian Broadcasting Corporation television network's evening news (*Dagsrevyen*, NRK, 12 December 2012) immediately following this, he said he believed he could get even better, that he could improve in all areas:

> I make mistakes all the time and it is human to make mistakes. But it's still possible to weed out many of the mistakes, and with time, play with even greater precision. And in general, I still have a lot to learn about chess. It is such a rich game that one will never master it entirely.

The challenges for mental health care services

These principles can be applied in the field of mental health care. There are, however, a number of reasons why this approach has a hard time gaining a foothold within mental health care services, and it's worth taking a moment to address these reasons in further detail.

A while back, I met with a man who had taken part in group counselling at one of Norway's psychiatric hospitals. He told me that on several occasions in the course of his treatment he had filled out a self-report questionnaire about his symptoms. We decided to write to the hospital and ask for his journal, so we could look at the results together. It turned out that when he started with group counselling he reported many symptoms and thus that he was feeling very poorly. Halfway through the treatment, he was asked to fill out the questionnaire again. He responded the same this time as he had when he started; in other words, he saw no improvement. His treatment, nonetheless, continued as before without any change. When his treatment was officially completed, he filled out the questionnaire again with the same result. The man's experience was that the treatment hadn't helped, and the therapists at the hospital were informed of this. Instead of taking this into account and coming up with other ways of helping him, he was offered another round of the same treatment. In other words, they believed there was nothing wrong with the treatment, but that the problem was with the man's ability to benefit from it. After taking part in the first two sessions of the second round, he dropped out. The final report from the hospital concluded that he was not especially motivated.

Within mental health care services, there is not much tradition of actively implementing clients' feedback when designing services. The outcomes, the real impact of the treatment, are usually evaluated by the professionals themselves. Unfortunately, these assessments are not very reliable. Whether it comes through self-report questionnaires or other input channels, we do not take sufficient account of the feedback we receive from clients, particularly when the results are negative.

Mental health care is a field largely controlled by a meritocracy (that is, an underlying philosophy that those who appear to have the greatest ability and achievements, as well as extending the greatest effort should reap the greatest rewards), a clear professional structure, and a knowledge hierarchy. At the top of this organizational chart sits the natural sciences' view of knowledge, which is espoused by the psychiatrists and, to a certain extent, the psychologists. This knowledge is generally unchallenged, as it is specialized knowledge that gives its proponents the authority to define practice. Psychologists in Norway have succeeded in taking charge of mental health care. In many areas, they have received the same authority as psychiatrists and thus achieved a comparable position of authority. There is, however, cause to ask whether this has benefited the clients. Psychologists seldom challenge the existing knowledge paradigm, preferring instead to uphold it along with their own credibility. In fact, one of the most problematic aspects of the mental health care field is the unilateral support of the status quo in terms of approaches to mental health care. There are powerful forces and interests invested in maintaining the existing paradigm, because it also secures the legitimacy of professionals. In order for feedback from clients to have an impact, psychiatrists and psychologists must relinquish a certain amount of control. Professionals must be willing to adapt their approach to identify the best way to help each individual.

The time has come for a new format

Changes are taking place. In pioneering institutions throughout Norway and the other Scandinavian countries, client feedback is being heard and services developed accordingly. They achieve impressive results, but these institutions are also vulnerable. When they make changes in accordance with client feedback, they often no longer fit in – neither with the prevailing view of mental health care nor with centrally imposed organizational models. It is therefore time to change the format: we can't adjust client feedback to suit professionals' expert understanding. It is the professionals and their services that must change.

The mental health care services we have today are too often like an old WAP phone. You can make outgoing calls, receive incoming calls, and send text messages on a very small screen, but the users want something else. They want the Internet with access to flexible, comprehensive services, where they personally take part in designing the content. Many service providers have understood this, so they try to force the Internet into the old mobile phone with the outdated format. Mental health care providers are doing everything they can to get the users to like the old mobile phone, but the majority don't want it. They want the new solutions in a new format. They want a smartphone.

We can develop our own version of "smartphone" services that respond to users' feedback about what constitutes good help, and we have to begin with ourselves. Gandhi said, "Be the change you want to see in the world." As a therapist you can develop in concert with the client feedback, and you will discover sides of both yourself and your profession that you've never seen before.

5

IMPROVING AS A THERAPIST

It is not that I'm so smart. But I stay with the questions much longer.
Albert Einstein

My grandmother's coleslaw

My grandmother grew up in Hemnes in the county of Nordland, in Norway. When she was a little girl, her mother died and her Aunt Anna took over the custody and care of her and her five siblings. They were all very fond of Aunt Anna. She made sure the siblings received a good upbringing, in spite of their mother's premature death, and also used the family's network to ensure that each and every one of them received some education. Aunt Anna was manager of the telegraph office in Hemnes and a brilliant role model for the coming generation.

When my grandmother was 17 years old, she moved to the home of her uncle in Askvoll in western Norway. He was an apothecary, and

Grandmother worked for him for several years. Later in her life, she would often talk about this as a time when she was happy and learned a good deal. When she came to visit Hemnes during her vacations, she had nice dresses, coat, shoes and bracelets that the girls in Hemnes had never seen before. Grandmother was a pretty girl and was admired by many.

During one of these visited she met my grandfather. He was 12 years older than she was and general manager of the margarine factory in the neighbouring village of Finneidfjord. They were married in 1937, when Grandmother was 22 years old. That same year, my grandfather built the large house that would be my childhood home. It has been described as the nicest house in Sør-Rana at that time and, in the common vernacular, it was called "Lille Skaugum". My grandmother and grandfather had a bathroom with tiles, a water closet, parquet floors, and central heating. Grandmother brought with her lovely fabrics from Bergen, out of which she sewed bedding and tablecloths. It was not possible to buy such things ready-made at that time.

In spite of this prosperity, the post-war period was still a time of financial hardship for my grandparents. They had three sons, but it was not a given that all of them could pursue higher education. Grandmother thought education was very important and wanted her sons to receive the best possible education. She had not finished middle school herself. There are no living relatives who know the reason for this. Grandmother was extremely reluctant to speak about it. The subject was simply a passed over in silence.

Long before my father, the eldest of the sons, was going to start high school, she found a solution for their financial difficulties. At that time there was no high school nearby, so my father had to travel to Steinkjer and live in a small studio apartment, which was expensive. Grandmother therefore started up the production of mayonnaise and coleslaw. At the margarine factory where Grandfather was general manager, there was a vacant room that Grandmother was allowed to use. She had to buy a large mixer, and it's likely she borrowed money to manage this. My father described how large quantities of egg and oil were stirred together in the mixer and finally a strip of coloured power that disappeared into the mixture. The mayonnaise was put into jars, and the boys helped out with pasting on the labels. To make a salad, they had to grate carrots and cabbage. A large tray with a knife on a slant like a slicer in the middle of the tray was set up between two chairs. They pushed the cabbage back and forth as the shreddings tumbled down into a large vat below.

Distribution of fresh food was not very easy at that time. For that reason, the margarine factories were spread all over the country and Grandmother had the same idea about the mayonnaise and the salad. The salad was sold to shops by the bucket and she sent along paper cups so that the salad could be weighed out in the shop. The mayonnaise was sold by the jar throughout northern Norway, and her customers included large commissions for the military. The boys helped with the production, but Grandmother had also hired two local women. She worked on this enterprise in the evenings, when she had no other work tasks. She did all the books herself and kept the orders organized. Grandmother was clever with such things, and my father remembers the books spread out across the living room table. Together with my grandfather, she set up a joint-stock company and ran the production like a regular business.

At some point after my father finished high school, Grandfather apparently decided enough was enough and that the two younger brothers would have to make do with a little less education, but Grandmother put her foot down and insisted that there would be no stopping their education here. So, production continued until all the boys finished high school. When Grandmother had accomplished this, she could shut down with satisfaction. She was bored producing mayonnaise and salad. It reminded her too much of housework and over time became a tedious obligation. Still, she never gave up along the way. She continued until she had accomplished what she'd set out to do, to give her sons the education she herself had not had.

Success is not about being among the lucky few who are born with talent or special abilities. It is neither solely about hard work, something many of us do throughout our entire lives without necessarily leading to improvement. However, when you ask why some people are successful, the proffered explanation is often natural talent or hard work. In such books as *Talent is Overrated* by Geoff Colvin (2008), *Outliers* by Malcolm Gladwell (2008), and *The Talent Code* by Daniel Coyle (2009), however, we find another explanation for what makes some people extremely adept within their field. These authors were all inspired by K.A. Ericsson's concept of deliberate practice, but put into a context that applies to all of us.

In this chapter, we translate the knowledge about deliberate practice to apply to you as a therapist. You need not have an innate talent to be a really good therapist; there are other important mechanisms. Improving or achieving something requires a specific type of mindset. My grandmother did not have any particular talent for commercial food preparation, but she knew what she wanted and took advantage of the resources that were available to her. She had a mindset that said she would manage this, even though sometimes she found it boring. She also took chances with no guarantee of success. We will start by looking at what research tells us about mindsets.

Mindsets

Carol Dweck is a professor of psychology at Stanford University and one of the world's leading researchers on personality, motivation, and development. She has developed a theory based on the principle that it is not only our abilities or talents that determine whether we will achieve success but the attitude with which we approach our goals. As a young researcher, Dweck observed something that would change her life. She was interested in finding out how people handled setbacks. Through her research she observed how children reacted to difficult tasks. She brought the children into the room, made sure they were comfortable, and then gave them tasks to solve. The tasks began simply and became increasingly difficult. She observed the children's reactions to the tasks, how they solved the problems and overcame the challenges. Then she saw something unexpected. Faced with a difficult task a 10-year-old boy tugged at his hair, rubbed his hands together, smacked his lips, and burst out, "I love a challenge!" Another boy who was sweating over the task looked up with a satisfied expression and said, "You know, I hoped this would be educational."

These reactions astonished Dweck. She believed that either you can handle adversity or you can't. She didn't think that anyone would love adversity. Since that time, these children have been Dweck's role models. The children understood that human characteristics, such as intellectual skills, can be improved through effort. It was not just that they didn't become discouraged in the face of adversity; they didn't even experience it as adversity. They viewed it as a learning opportunity.

Through her research, Dweck has seen how our self-image and character traits have a strong impact on how we live our lives. If we think our character traits are written in stone and that there is little we can do to improve them, we have what Dweck calls a *fixed mindset* (Dweck, 2006). We think that the way we are born defines how we will always be and that there is not much to be done about it. Thus, we will continually try to prove that we are good enough and evaluate ourselves all the time. Our success becomes the definition of who we are, and there are many worries connected to constantly having to perform well enough. People with a growth mindset, on the other hand, believe that the qualities we have were given at birth are just a starting point for development. Even though people are born with different personalities and temperaments, we think that everyone can change and grow through experience. People with such an emotional mindset may not believe that everyone can become everything they might want to become, but they do believe that a person's true potential is unknown. It is not possible to foresee what practice and commitment can achieve.

People with a growth mindset will appreciate difficult tasks and not be afraid of making mistakes. They view making mistakes as a natural part of life and development and don't think their mistakes define who they are. A person with a fixed mindset will feel a constant need to prove their worth and that it's important not to make mistakes, because that would imply that they aren't good enough.

In an experiment, Dweck gave 330 schoolchildren between 11 and 12 years of age a questionnaire to find out what they thought about talent and about intelligence in particular. The children who believed that intelligence was something constant that could not be changed were put into the fixed mindset group. The children who thought that intelligence could be developed through effort were put into the growth mindset group. The children then received a series of exercises, the first eight of which were quite simple and the next four very difficult. As the children were struggling with their challenges, Dweck observed two different patterns. The children in the fixed mindset group quickly began to run down their own abilities and blame it on intelligence when they failed to find a solution for an exercise. They would say things like "I guess I'm not very smart", "I have such a poor memory", or "I'm no good at this kind of exercise". What was striking was that these children had succeeded in solving many of the exercises to begin with, and both their intelligence and memory had functioned perfectly fine. As soon as problems arose, however, they lost faith in their intelligence. Two-thirds of them showed a decline in strategic problem-solving, and more than half began using completely ineffectual strategies.

Did the children in the growth mindset group blame their lack of intelligence when they met with difficulties? Dweck found that they did not place blame on anything. They did not focus on finding explanations for why they failed; in fact, they did not consider adversity to be a failure in any sense at all. Within this group, 80% improved the quality of their problem-solving strategies when faced with the difficult exercises, and one-quarter of the group actually performed better. They taught themselves new strategies for solving the difficult exercises, and a few solved problems that they initially thought were too difficult. Even though at the outset they didn't have better abilities than the fixed mindset group, they ended up demonstrating much better performances. This had nothing to do with intelligence or motivation. On the contrary, Dweck made sure that everyone was equally motivated. What distinguished them was the way they thought about themselves and their abilities.

In 2006, Shizuka Arakawa won the gold medal in figure skating at the Winter Olympics. She was then 24 years old and had been training since she was five. Winning a gold medal requires a flawless performance of movements that seem impossible for the rest of us. Perfecting such movements requires years of practice and a lot of falling down. For Arakawa, it took 19 years. A study of figure skaters showed that sub-elite figure skaters spent a lot of time practising jumps they already knew how to do, while the very best figure skaters spent most of their time on jumps they had not yet mastered. The latter kind of practice is what leads to Olympic medals and involves many falls before mastery comes. Failure in figure skating implies falling on the ground, protected only by a thin suit against cold, hard ice. Arakawa's road to the gold medal involved at least 20,000 falls on the ice, but they produced results. Her story is impressive in its own right, but is also a wonderful metaphor. Falling on one's behind 20,000 times produces great performances.

Therapists want to improve

It perhaps sounds trite, but most therapists choose this profession because they want to help people. When somebody asks us why we want to work in this field, it's not about money and fame. We want to make a difference in people's lives and work at something meaningful. When therapists describe what it's like to work with clients, they use words such as "interesting", "fascinating", "rewarding", "meaningful", "stimulating", and "exciting." Some view it as a privilege. It represents a part of life that therapists personally feel provides meaning and value.

In a comprehensive study, researchers David Orlinsky from the University of Chicago and Helge Rønnestad from the University of Oslo made an in-depth investigation of how therapists experience their work and professional development (Orlinsky & Rønnestad, 2005). Over a 15-year period, they collected detailed information from close to 5,000 psychotherapists with different career backgrounds, practice specialties, and theoretical approaches. When they analysed different aspects of being a therapist, they were able to identify two different ways that therapists approached work with clients. One of these is called *healing involvement*, characterized by the therapists experiencing themselves as being personally committed and confirming in relation to the client, showing a high degree of empathy, and communicating well. They have a feeling of effectiveness and can work constructively with problems as these arise. *Stressful involvement*, on the other hand, is a pattern in which therapists often experience difficulties in therapy and have less-than-constructive ways of handling these problems. They will thereby avoid becoming involved and experience a feeling of boredom or anxiety in the sessions with the client.

Orlinsky and Rønnestad identified three more conditions that led to therapists having an experience of healing involvement. The first was the experience of improvement over time, that they gradually bettered their therapeutic skills, experienced increased mastery, and little by little became more adept at doing what they had previously experienced as difficult. In other words, therapists like to believe that they improve over the years. Among the therapists, 86% reported that they were "highly motivated" to develop professionally, which is wholly exceptional. There is scarcely any other profession, as a group, that is so interested in becoming more proficient at what they do, and this interest continues throughout the entire career. The second thing that motivated therapists was theoretical breadth. The therapists who had an eclectic approach and who were not too attached to a particular method experienced a larger degree of healing involvement. Having a series of models for understanding a client's problems, as well as potential methods with which to address these problems, made it possible for the therapists to experience being useful more often and with more clients. The third and most powerful influence on therapists' experience of being helpful was manifested in palpable growth as a therapist. Therapists like to believe they are developing now, at this very moment. This motivates them to perform at their best for the clients and improves their work ethic. It contributes to professional reflection, which in turn motivates them to seek out courses, guidance, and fresh input by reading literature in their field. What gives therapists the greatest feeling of growth here and now, however, is the quality of the encounter with the clients. The therapists think that they develop the most in the meeting with the clients, not through seminars or books. It is actually the case that therapists think that the clients are their best teachers.

The biggest limitation of Orlinsky and Rønnestad's study is that it does not consider whether there is any connection between the therapists' development and clinical effectiveness. Although several factors that increase both healing involvement and stressful involvement have been identified, there are no indications of the connection between these factors and the therapists' outcomes. A more recent study by Daryl Chow (2014) found that therapists who reported a high level of healing involvement in clinical practice actually had a greater likelihood of scoring poorly when it came to the clients' outcomes.

In spite of good intentions and commitment to one's work, it is not always easy to be a therapist. We are constantly told to learn the most recent methods and follow recommended guidelines, which allegedly are to ensure the quality of treatment. Many therapists can also experience fear if they do not constantly seek out and apply the latest recommended methods. If we carry out our practice in flexible or non-traditional ways, according to the wishes of the client, we can risk being told that we are not practising "correct therapy" and that this is unethical. The current version of correct therapy is evidence-based practice which has been subject to examination through sufficient RCT studies. The problems with this were discussed in Chapter 2. In addition, therapists often face endless and oppressive paper work, idiotic production requirements, and a variety of obligatory registration and mapping tasks – requirements that hinder rather than help anybody to be the good therapist they so want to be. In spite of this, there are some therapists who achieve exceedingly good results, which demonstrates that it is fully possible to improve over the years. However, the road to improvement starts by ascertaining how one is performing here and now. Realistically this is something very few therapists actually do. Let us look more closely at how we evaluate ourselves.

Large differences in the outcomes of respective therapists

Outcomes achieved by different therapists tend to vary dramatically. It seems the best therapists are successful with approximately 70% of their clients, the worst with only about 20%. The therapist effect explains most of the differences in therapy outcomes, far more than the therapeutic approach. In clinics, some therapists are more effective than others, regardless of which method they use. As a person seeking help, in other words, the particular therapist plays a more important part than the method employed in working towards a positive therapeutic outcome.

Further, findings show that, regardless of whether or not they achieve good outcomes, therapists are not particularly adept at identifying the clients who do not experience change. In one study by Hannan and his colleagues (2005), researchers wanted to determine how proficient therapists were at evaluating whether the clients experienced a worsening of their condition. The therapists' assessments were compared with assessments made using a statistical method. The therapists were familiar with the purpose of the study, familiar with the outcome scale that was used, and informed that it was likely that 8% would experience worsening. Nonetheless, the therapists were able to identify worsening in only one out of 550 clients. In other words, the therapists failed to notice the deterioration in 39 of 40 clients, which was the actual number of clients whose condition worsened. By comparison, the statistical method was able to identify 36 out of 40. The therapists' evaluation also determined that the condition of 91% was improved by the treatment, even though the actual number was less than half (40%).

It appears that many of us suffer from what has been called the "Lake Wobegon effect". In his weekly radio programme *A Prairie Home Companion*, Garrison Keillor reported from the fictional city of Lake Wobegon, Minnesota, "where all the women are strong, all the men are good-looking, and all the children are above average." Named for this town, the Lake Wobegon effect describes a natural human tendency to overestimate one's own proficiency.

Walfish, McAlister, O'Donnell, and Lambert (2012) asked 129 therapists to assess their own abilities in a study originally submitted with the title "Are all psychotherapists from Lake Wobegon? An investigation of self-assessment bias in mental health providers". One-quarter of the therapists claimed that they were at the top level and performed better than 90% of their colleagues. On average, the therapists assessed themselves as being 80% better than their colleagues, while only 8.4% believed their ranking to be less than 75%. Nobody assessed themselves as below average. It can perhaps be viewed as positive that we have such healthy self-confidence, but in principle such an understanding of own abilities makes improvement unlikely. It is difficult to know where you're going when you don't know where you are.

In Chapter 4 we addressed K.A. Ericsson's research, which showed that, when learning a new skill, one achieves an acceptable level quickly, but often remains at that plateau. Therapists are no different. Repeated studies examining the differences in therapy outcomes do not show that experience as a determining factor. How long you have been working as a therapist has little impact on your outcomes. However, it may not be so strange that we don't improve over the years when we have such high opinions of ourselves, as the study by Walfish et al. (2012) demonstrated. A pianist might hear dissonance when he strikes the wrong note and will thus know where he needs to improve. Unfortunately, therapists don't always appear to hear the dissonances, and we therefore don't know what we are supposed to improve.

We may also believe that we are improving when, in fact, we are not. Our evaluation of own performance is basically unreliable as well as too often inaccurate. The problem is this kind of mindset gets in the way of our development as individual therapists and the development of the profession as a whole. Paradoxically, most therapists do indeed want to improve, but without reliable feedback on one's own performance this becomes virtually impossible. However, with the right approach to practice, it is possible to improve over time. Let us first look at the research to see what the best therapists do that separates them from the rest of us.

What separates the best therapists from the rest?

When Daryl Chow was a PhD student at Curtin University in Australia, he researched what makes some therapists extremely proficient. Originally from Singapore, he started his career as a psychologist at the country's only psychiatric hospital and worked there for a number of years. He and his colleagues became interested in the use of feedback and conducted trials to investigate the use of ORS and SRS. They compared feedback with no feedback in studies similar to those Michael Lambert had already done, which I described in Chapter 3. Chow was interested in these comparisons and in how the individual therapists applied the feedback. In the trials, they saw large differences in the results for different therapists, but there were also differences in the degree to which the therapists were able to make use of the feedback.

I came into contact with Chow after Scott Miller recommended that I speak with him. Chow has collaborated with Miller for many years, and they exchanged ideas about underlying principles for Chow's doctoral work.

In a Skype conversation, Chow told me that initially he was not specifically interested in research but was satisfied that he finished his training as a psychologist. Still, this issue interested him so much that he had to pursue the questions he and Miller had discussed. When the opportunity presented itself to attain a PhD at Curtin University, he and his wife packed up their belongings and moved to Perth. Chow is one of the few researchers in the world investigating what therapists who achieve the best outcomes do that sets them apart from the rest.

Chow's first challenge was to connect with enough therapists within the same organization who had received feedback on a regular basis about the progress of clients. In Great Britain, he found Bill Andrews in a network of 69 therapists who had been routinely using formal feedback for many years. First, Chow analysed the data from all 69 therapists. Through here he gained access to a total of 4,580 clients. Chow wanted to find out whether there were differences in the outcomes of the therapists as other studies had shown. He also wanted to see whether there was any information that could explain the differences. A similar study had already been done by Okiishi, Lambert, Nielsen, and Ogles (2003). Chow more or less replicated this study (Chow, Miller, Seidel, Kane, & Thorntonet, 2015). Analyses of the 69 therapists showed that there were large differences between the therapists and that 5% of the variance could be explained by this therapist effect. This corresponded with earlier findings. Chow also investigated whether age, sex, years of experience, or professional or theoretical approach could explain the differences, but there was nothing that stood out.

Chow then went on to produce an extensive questionnaire that was sent to all the therapists. Together with Scott Miller, he identified what they wanted to investigate. A large portion of the material came from Ericsson's research on expertise and performance excellence. As in the violin study from Berlin described in Chapter 4, they were asked how much time they spent on different activities related to own professional development. Chow also had questions taken from Dweck's (2006) research on mindset, from social psychology, and from Orlinsky and Rønnestad's (2005) research on therapists. There were also questions about use of formal feedback in therapy. Of the 69 questionnaires that went out to the therapists, Chow received 17 responses that comprised the selection for the second study. These constituted a distorted selection because the majority of those who answered were the therapists with the best outcomes. However, there were some in the middle and some who had poor outcomes. Analysis of these 17 responses produced a therapist variable of 4–5%, which corresponded with previous findings.

Out of everything the therapists answered questions about, there was very little that stood out as significant in explaining the differences between them. The amount of time the therapists spent on solitary practice to improve their therapeutic skills, however, was a significant predictor for the results. This finding corresponds with the role of deliberate practice in the development of expertise as explained in the last chapter. What distinguished the best from the second best in the violin study from Berlin was solitary practice. Chow's study shows that this type of practice is also important among therapists.

The second significant finding involved feedback and the ways in which the therapists understood it. Here, also, not much appeared significant, except for the number of times the therapists were surprised by the feedback. The most effective therapists were more surprised with the feedback than the less effective. This might indicate that they are more open and more willing to accept feedback and take this as a signal that they should make adjustments.

Chow was also surprised by this finding. It suggested that the most effective therapists have qualities such as openness, receptiveness, and willingness to accept negative and positive feedback. Chow recommended a study by Najavits and Strupp (1994), which found that effective therapists were more self-critical and reported making more mistakes than the less effective therapists. In a more recent study (Nissen-Lie, Monsen, & Rønnestad, 2010), the therapists' self-doubt had a positive effect on how the clients assessed the alliance. Combined, these studies may indicate willingness on the part of the most effective therapists to evaluate their own contribution to the process and find ways to correct themselves and improve their performance. In Chow's study, "surprised by the clients' feedback" was negatively correlated with the therapists' assessment of healing involvement.

Further, Chow explained that the finding can also be explained by something called the "hypercorrection effect" (Metcalfe & Finn, 2011). This means that errors made with a high level of self-confidence are more likely to be corrected after being pointed out through feedback than errors made with little self-confidence. The discrepancy between what the therapist had expected and the feedback may prompt the hypercorrection effect. Accordingly, we pay more attention to unexpected feedback than to feedback that is expected.

While the therapist factor explains most of the variance in therapy, little research has been done on it. Hopefully, we will see more research like Chow's. Because he emphasizes that his study is only a preliminary study based on a small number of therapists, he is careful not to generalize too much. Through Ericsson's research on expertise and performance excellence, we can still implement the principles of deliberate practice in our development as therapists, because an abundance of research has demonstrated the efficacy of this type of practice in other disciplines.

This is how you can become one of the best

Acquiring feedback is only the beginning of becoming a better therapist. Once we incorporate feedback into our practice through repetition and reflection, we both learn something and improve our performance over time. We don't improve as a therapist simply by memorizing a handbook or learning special techniques that we can then employ in relation to clients. Improvement in the true sense is more about a disposition, understanding of learning, and refined performance which is more dynamic. We never know in advance what will produce the best outcome. Through trial and error, we will eventually develop the knowledge required to achieve excellent results. There are some elements which will help along the way.

Access to results

First of all, you must have access to your results, and you should create a system for these. You can read more about your outcomes in Chapter 3. Systematic feedback from your clients about whether or not they are experiencing improvement will tell you a great deal about whether you are successful as a therapist. Our own assessment of our performance is not accurate – remember the Lake Wobegon effect. You need more concrete facts. However, a study done by the Dutch researcher Kim de Jong, van Sluis, Nugter, Heiser, and Spinhoven (2012) showed that feedback is a complex process. They found that therapists did not always use feedback even when confronted with it. Therapists with higher self-efficacy, who believe they can solve problems and reach goals on their own, had a higher probability of deriving benefits from the feedback. Therapists with an attitude of openness to feedback achieved more rapid improvement with their clients.

To create a system for reviewing outcomes you can use a computer program that facilitates tabulating the feedback you receive from your clients. This can provide a good overview of which clients you are succeeding with and who is not improving. In all likelihood, you will begin to see a pattern in the results and thereby be able to identify issues or areas where you regularly encounter challenges. From there, it will be easier to know where you need to improve and what you already do well.

It can help our self-confidence to understand what we do well, but what will really improve your performance as a therapist is more practice in the areas where the results are not as good. Remember the best figure skaters, who practised the jumps they had not yet mastered. This meant they fell on their behinds a lot, but it also led to their winning Olympic medals.

Find a mentor/the dependable coach

I have had many supervisors over the years, but few I could call mentors. Luckily, I found a mentor at my first job. Andy Huggins at the Hagen treatment unit in Norway has been a pioneer in the use of feedback in therapy. Andy took a fledgling, recent graduate psychologist under his wing and showed me the complicated nature of the profession. I accompanied Andy on home visits, school meetings, and conversations with families and networks. I saw how Andy did things, and in time was made the lead therapist in various sessions. We were working with difficult sets of problems, since Hagen was an institution of last resort. Andy gave me feedback on how I came across in the sessions with families. Combined with the feedback from the families themselves, this enabled me to understand how I needed to develop in order to achieve better outcomes. Working with Andy at the start gave me a sense of security, but gradually I became more independent and did things on my own. If I got stuck, I could always go back to Andy and discuss what I'd experienced. Andy had wise words and helpful suggestions, but always emphasized that the feedback I got from the clients was the most important. I caught myself saying: "As Andy used to say… " many times after I left Hagen.

There is a strong tradition of supervision in mental health services, which is considered to be psychotherapy's signature pedagogy. Few studies of the effect of supervision on results have been done, and those that do exist provide limited empirical support for the claim that supervision is more effective than other types of training, even though many therapists will give supervision a high ranking (Watkins, 2010, 2011). In order to justify the extensive amount of time spent on supervision, it must also benefit the clients. When you find a supervisor, you must first and foremost be sure that this individual wants to hear about your outcomes. A supervisor who is not interested in outcomes will never be able to help you improve. Imagine if Marit Bjørgen's coach had not been concerned about whether she came in first or not. As long as she held her ski poles correctly, her times were not all that important? No, I don't think so.

Further, you need a supervisor whom you trust. The relationship with the supervisor is important because you must dare to fail with your supervisor. As we now know, a large part of improvement hinges on the ability to notice where we fall on our faces. The learner–supervisor relationship must be such that it's possible to show mistakes and shortcomings. At the same time, both must recognize that everything is a learning experience, that mistakes are opportunities to do better next time. As we have learned from Dweck's (2006) research, the supervisor must be interested in your work investment as a therapist. Gaining an overview of outcomes helps you to understand where you have room for improvement, but it is not a static definition of you as a therapist. You can always improve once you recognize what isn't helping.

Your supervisor needs to know a lot about the particular sphere in which you are working. A football coach isn't much use to a handball team. They even have specialized coaches for goalkeepers. Just because an individual has acquired a certain level of supervisor status does not mean that they can be a supervisor for just anything. The supervisor must know more than you within your specialized area, so that he or she can challenge you when you get stuck. They must help you acquire a larger repertoire of approaches and give you corrections or suggestions for how you can do things differently. The supervisor must see what you are unable to see for yourself, and must recognize where your approach falls short and where it works.

Set clear, defined goals and practice

Practise one thing at a time. Don't imagine you are going to master all kinds of issues right away. By choosing one spot to focus, you can practise more. When you see variations on the same theme time after time, you will ultimately master this issue at a level that is far above average. You will have built up a rich repertoire of alternative approaches and can then act more directly in response to what the client presents in that moment. The best therapists have a deeper, more accessible, and more nuanced knowledge about the specific sets of problems they are working with. Thus, they can relate to the clients in many different ways in order to ensure the best possible outcome.

Robbie Babbins-Wagner, head of the Calgary Counseling Centre, explains how she focused on a single type of clinical population up until she had mapped out every potential characteristic of the issue (Babbins-Wagner, 2017). She met with client after client, based on the idea that, if you are going to become really good at something, you can't address a broad array of different problems. She met 50, 100, or 200 clients with depression or physical abuse in close relationships, and she gradually saw common patterns that she otherwise would have missed. For example, when she was working on spousal abuse, she learned that, even if the violence ended and the couple was doing better, a relapse would almost always occur. Since she was aware of this pattern, she was ready for it and did not view it as unsuccessful therapy or the end of the treatment, rather as a predictable stumbling block along the way that had to be overcome.

When you monitor your outcomes over time, you will gradually understand where improvements are needed. You can also expand your field of expertise as you gradually come to master one type of issue thoroughly.

Trying, failing, reflection, and increased knowledge

We receive feedback all the time. Our clients try to give us information beyond the systematic feedback we request from them. We get it from collaborating partners and from the families of those we are working to help. But even though we can become proficient at receiving feedback, this does not mean that we know how to use it or how we can incorporate it into our practice over time. On the contrary, we can develop habits that allow us to avoid facing the feedback we receive. We can explain it away as being irrelevant or convince ourselves that the feedback helps neither us nor our clients. Learning to employ feedback is something completely different from simply receiving it. When you become skilled at implementing feedback, you will experience actual improvement. In turn, this reinforces your belief that paying attention to feedback is beneficial.

The secret to improvement is to have conscious control over what you are practising. Compelling yourself not to function on autopilot will help you avoid ending up at a level that is "good enough". Taking active and deliberate control of your actions will raise your performance level and lead to improvement. Feedback comes in different forms and from different quarters. Some might be concrete, such as suggestions for alternative approaches from the clients, your supervisor, or your superior. When you receive this type of feedback, it's important to test it as soon as possible. Don't be concerned about what you think of it or indulge in a long round of reflections about its immediate usefulness. Try it out, preferably several times. It can often be tempting to reflect upon and discuss the feedback, but often this will interfere with your actions. Instead, give it a try first, and then, on the basis of that experience, you will have something to reflect upon. If you're hung up on the feedback, you may avoid actually practising with an aim of improvement. It is premature to reflect on the feedback before you have tested it. The outcome you achieve by implementing is what counts. This will become a process of trial and error where you will have a lot of time to try things out and enough time to reflect upon the outcome of your efforts (Lemow, Woolway, & Yezzi, 2012). Using feedback is about implementing it in real life, about actually changing the way you do things. Reflection over what you have done is an essential part of achieving an upward learning curve.

However, not all feedback gives you clear approach options. Feedback on outcomes in therapy, for example, tells you whether you or not you have succeeded but not what you can do if you get stuck. In such cases, you might discuss this with your clients and with a supervisor to formulate ideas for what can be done differently. You can arrive at new approaches in conversation with others, but those who perform best in their field also spend a lot of time on acquiring more knowledge on their own. We saw this in Daryl Chow, Miller, Seidel, et al.'s (2015) research, and in great performances in other disciplines. If you have questions or are baffled by something, try to figure it out by yourself. Read books, read articles, or call somebody who can help you with what you're trying to solve. You will not improve by simply soliciting feedback on a day-to-day basis. You must reflect upon the results between sessions, carry out measures to expand your scope as a therapist, and find new ways of relating to your clients, especially when you hit the wall. It is what you do *before and after* the therapy sessions that brings about improvement, not simply what you do *in* the therapy sessions.

There are no shortcuts to becoming a good therapist, and there is no a handbook or user guide that can tell you what you must do to succeed in every instance. Becoming really good at something is more about your attitude and mindset regarding learning and performance. Thus, you should not be concerned about being clever. Failing or making mistakes, without shame, can provide increased motivation for learning. The most effective therapists more talk about errors and are more critical of their own practice. Setting your sights on being flawless leads to worse results, and you may end up seeking out fewer challenging work assignments. Normalizing your own mistakes will make it easier to try out new approaches, because both you and the clients are aware that, in the end, if you want to achieving the best possible result will require some amount of trial and error.

> *Ever tried. Ever failed. No matter. Try again. Fail again. Fail better.*
> Samuel Beckett

Reflections from a therapist who actually improved

While we believe may we are improving as therapists in each meeting with our clients, it's hard to know if this is true if we do not get feedback on the results. Do you remember Morten Anker's couples therapy study in Chapter 3? Ten therapists took part in the study. Nine of these improved after they started soliciting feedback. However, the effect of feedback on the therapists varied. The least effective (those with the poorest outcomes without feedback) benefited the most from feedback compared with the most effective therapists. In fact, one of the therapists who had the poorest results at the beginning was the therapist with the best results after receiving feedback. She described her progress as involving becoming more direct and courageous, and feeling safe in the knowledge that her clients would teach her what to do when she was not helping. She also described learning about how client progress is a shared responsibility (Anker, Duncan, & Sparks, 2009).

The gifts required to be a good therapist are not necessarily innate. It is often said that people who are very good at something "possess a special talent for it", or "that it comes very naturally to them". However, when you talk to people who are very good at something, they say that talent is responsible for only a very small part of their results and the rest is practice, practice, practice. It's the same for therapists. Being a proficient therapist is not static; rather, your investment will always have an impact on the result. If you have had good results for a period of time and then sit back and think that now you can manage this well without any particular effort, there is no guarantee of achieving good results with the next person you try to help.

Moments that change you

Have you ever experienced a moment that moved you profoundly and changed your way of thinking? I have. When I was a teenager, I had a chat with my mother. I wondered if it wasn't difficult to work with people who were going through hard times. Didn't she feel sorry for them? My mother responded that she never felt sorry for people; she could feel for them, but she didn't feel sorry for them. She explained that as soon as you start feeling sorry for somebody you make them pitiful and diminish them. In a way you deprive them of the right to retain their dignity in the midst of all their difficulties. When you feel sorry for people, you also become concerned about rescuing them. You cast yourself in the role of a hero. No, my mother would never do that. While she was concerned about helping people, she also had expectations that they would have resources and opportunities through which they could improve their own situation. My mother thought that first and foremost they had to help themselves, because she believed that all people have an inherent ability to influence their own lives. "So, I don't feel sorry for people, Birgit, but I can feel for them," she often said. And that made all the difference. This is a lesson I continue to carry with me in life and the basis upon which I always work. Not because I read somewhere that that is how I should work, but because I sense inside me that it is right. It has become a part of me.

Some people are more easily influenced than others. They take in new information and new experiences openly and with a sense of wonder. Remember the research of Kim de Jong et al. (2012), which I presented earlier in this chapter, and Daryl Chow, who found in his study that the most effective therapists were more surprised about negative feedback. In order to improve as a therapist, both acquiring and applying feedback is wholly essential. Some therapists appear to master this better than others. Although we have not yet identified exactly what makes it easier for some people to benefit from feedback than others, it appears that openness to the feedback is important. This can lead to gathering more information, which in turn will lead to trying out new approaches, and ultimately that your performance as a therapist will change.

How much can we actually influence our own development and success in working life? We interact with superiors and colleagues who will influence the choices we make, and we are exposed to a large number of circumstances over which we have no control. Still, the research of Professor Richard Wiseman (2003) from the University of Hertfordshire in England shows that luck can be influenced to a certain degree. He started investigating whether people considered themselves to be lucky or unlucky. His findings showed that approximately 50% considered themselves lucky, 36% neither lucky nor unlucky, and 14% said that were consistently unlucky. Wiseman subsequently tried to determine what really differentiated the groups. He found that the lucky ones were more open to possibilities (or learning) that arise spontaneously, while those who considered themselves to be unlucky were more creatures of habit who fixated more on specific types of results. In social situations, for example, the unlucky people tended interact with people who were like themselves. Lucky people on the other hand would be more open to meeting people by chance. Lucky people also smiled twice as much, attracted others to a larger degree, and increased the probability of random and varied meetings. Opportunities that arise by chance benefit those who are open to them. Wiseman found out that establishing and maintaining a network of luck characterized a type of behaviour that played an important role in achieving success, something the lucky ones were especially good at. This was Wiseman's main finding: we can create our own luck. He discovered that being in the right place at the right time was actually about having the right mindset.

This brings us back to Dweck's (2006) research on motivation and mindsets. Although we can be internally motivated to improve, this doesn't mean that it's an innate ability. On the contrary, it can be learned. Wiseman took his research a step further and explained the main principles of lucky behaviour to the group that considered itself to be unlucky. He also taught them some specific techniques. After they had tried out these exercises for a month, they reported back to Wiseman. The results were dramatic: 80 were happier and more satisfied with life – and luckier.

A person can change their attitude to both learning and performance on their own. However, this is largely contingent upon being part of an organization that values this type of thinking and that encourages and supports the growth and development of therapists in the workplace. Growing in the field of mental health care as an individual therapist is difficult. The strength found in a supportive organization is possible. The next chapter examines this further.

6

IMPROVING THE ORGANIZATION

Dream more than others think practical.
Expect more than others think possible.
Care more than others think wise.

Howard Schultz

LEGO turns failure into success

Founded in 1932 by the Dane Ole Kirk Christiansen, the LEGO Company started out as a small carpentry shop. Today the company name is synonymous with their line of plastic building bricks, introduced in 1958 and now the most popular toy in the world. Everyone has a relationship to LEGO, from the gas station we played with in the 1970s to the Star Wars space ships our own children play with today. It hardly seems possible that a company with products so beloved by so many generations could run into problems, but in 2003 it did. Sales dropped by 35% in the USA and 29% globally, and one year later they experienced their greatest downturn ever. With massive debt and on the brink of bankruptcy, the family-owned company might have been easy prey for a larger corporation. Miraculously, LEGO managed to pull itself up by its bootstraps. In the subsequent years the company managed to reverse its losses into profits and now ranks third worldwide in toy sales. (Robertson & Breen, 2013).

Jørgen Vig Knudstorp saved LEGO from ruin. He was hired in 2001 and promoted to CEO in 2004. One of LEGO's main problems was that it had overextended itself. Knudstorp saw that the company needed a completely new paradigm, but did not want to implement extensive downsizing measures that were likely to do more harm than good. Among his first acts was travel to Virginia in the USA to attend BrickFest, an annual convention for adult LEGO fans. He came to learn what was special about LEGO: that it is a uniquely creative material, easy to assemble and harder to take apart. LEGO is ideal for teaching children how to think systematically and creatively. Knudstorp understood that the problem was not in the product itself but in the company's attempt to compete head-to-head with video games and lifestyle brands that were taking over the market. Through the launches of a clothing line, watches, and amusement parks, it had forgotten about the core enterprise. It was time to get back to basics (Robertson & Breen, 2013).

It sold off all the sideline enterprises that were not related to the core product. It was harder to change the attitude of the employees. Up until then, designers had relatively free rein when it had come to creating ever more imaginative figures. As a result, the models had become more complex, which required the company to come up with new components all the time. By 2004 the number of components had exploded from 7,000 to 12,400 in just seven years. Naturally, the costs had gone through the roof. However, an even greater cause for concern was that the new models did not interest children. The adults perhaps thought they were neat, but the youngsters could not stand them.

It was less the fault of the designers than the directors. They allowed the designers to do what they wanted in the name of innovation, which had the company headed for an innovative suicide. With Knudstorp at the helm, management introduced new guidelines for the staff. The entire culture had to change. Instead of being predominantly concerned with pursuing individual ideas, the focus had to shift towards the success of the company. That meant designers had to deliver results that enabled the company to earn money, not just manufacture products that they personally felt were exciting. Prior to launching a new product, they used children as experts and listened to their feedback in focus groups. The children noticed an incredible amount of detail and knew exactly what they wanted. By shifting attention to the wishes of the children, employees had to ask themselves all the time whether this was something the children would like and something they wanted more of (Robertson & Breen, 2013).

The field of mental health care can learn a lot from LEGO. After his first visit to BrickFest, Knudstorp began meeting regularly with adult LEGO fans, He understood how important customers' input was to saving the company. Some of the most enthusiastic fans were also involved in product development. Since that time, LEGO has actively encouraged its fans to suggest product ideas. The mental health care field needs a similar type of turnaround operation. Current feedback offers little cause for celebration, as outlined in Chapter 4, and many clients do attempt to speak up. The professionals within the field of mental health care have also developed a wide array of approaches and methods, not so different from the designers at LEGO. There is little context to the services being offered, and research communities around the world operate conscious of their own interests. A common objective appears impossible. The most important concern appears to be proving that the method under scrutiny is effective. The intentions may be good; the problem is that most methods will be found effective if sufficient money goes into researching them (as illustrated in Chapter 2). Finally, this research tells us little about what mental health problems are actually about. What is most worrisome about this approach is the complete failure to ask those who stands to benefit from it. There is no equal exchange of opinions between those who receive the help and those who are supposed to provide it. In this sense, the children in LEGO's focus group have a great deal to teach us.

When Knudstorp accepted the job of saving LEGO, he didn't do what many directors do to turn things around. He did not produce inspiring plans or hold passionate speeches for the staff about a better future. Instead, he attacked the overblown self-confidence of the employees and delivered a hard dose of reality. "We had to address the culture," Knudstorp said:

> We went through a painful process of berating ourselves and saying: You know what? There's no reason to be so enthusiastic. We don't have a brand that is as fantastic as we go around telling ourselves it is. We say that we do a lot for children's development, but we aren't selling very much, so how can that be true?
>
> (Robertson & Breen, 2013, p. 103)

Mental health care services need to go through the same painful process. This chapter will take a closer look at how to do this.

Can the field of mental health be turned around?

For private companies that sell products, profits are a matter of life or death. If LEGO doesn't sell its products, they will quite simply not survive. They are therefore compelled to be concerned about results. Mental health care services have a duty of care that ought to supersede profits. The services will always have customers, because aren't optional purchases, nor is there an endless supply of these types of services. People who are struggling psychologically have little choice but to accept the help offered locally. Nor do they have many options for investigating the quality of a service before receiving help. To be sure, the services are restructured on a regular basis, with an eye towards improvement, but that is just as much about cutting costs. Treatment services are seldom evaluated in terms of results. Is it then possible to adjust the mental health care services in accordance with what the population wants and information about what will help them?

During my first four years as a psychologist I worked at the treatment centre in Hagen and learned a lot. Ultimately, however, I had to move out into the world and explore how I might go about implementing what I had learned at Hagen in the context of a larger organization. When I read a job listing from the Stange area in 2009, I found the opportunity I had been waiting for. Stange was looking for a psychologist to take part in developing a mental health care service for children and families in the municipality, virtually from the ground up. I could not imagine a more perfect position. I was curious about how a mental health care service would appear if we developed it from scratch, based on the feedback we received from the families with whom we came into contact.

Another encouraging factor was that Kårhild Husom Løken was listed as the contact in the listing. I already knew about Kårhild because she had made a name for herself in the district for being particularly interested in the views of users and had been working for many years on user-perspective themes. She worked as a mental health care adviser and would be my most important collaborating partner. I knew she would be an ally, and that strengthened my conviction that Stange was right for me. It is extremely difficult to change established cultures. Knudstorp managed it, but he was the chief executive of the entire company. In Stange, on the other hand, we had the opportunity to build a culture from scratch, which is far simpler, but still requires discipline. If one doesn't take this work seriously from the beginning, cultures will emerge, particularly from employees and their previous experiences. This can occur very quickly and is an almost imperceptible process. Therefore, values and attitudes were our first priority when we started the work of planning the new service in Stange. From there, we could build the service one brick at a time.

How Starbucks built a company one cup at a time

In the summer of 2012, my husband and I took our children to Paris. We did all the typical tourist things. We went to the top of the Eiffel Tower, rode a boat down the Seine, visited Notre Dame, and strolled down Champs Élysées. Eventually we grew tired of all the walking and looked around for a place to rest. There were many charming sidewalk cafés to choose from, but where did you think we ended up? At Starbucks. I must admit it: I am a fan of Starbucks. We didn't have Starbucks in Norway then, so every time I was abroad it was lovely to sink down into one of their deep armchairs with a latte in my hand. Now my children love it too, and they make themselves at home there, stretching out on the couch. So what is it about Starbucks that draws people like me to these cafés? Starbucks emerged in response to feedback from customers.

The very first Starbucks café opened in Seattle in 1986 under the name "Il Giornale". The Starbucks company had been founded back in 1971 and consisted of retail stores that sold dark roast coffee beans from around the world and related appliances. When Howard Schultz, who would later become CEO, visited Starbucks for the first time in 1981, he had found his Mecca. Here he tasted coffee stronger than anything he had ever tasted before, and he had the feeling of having discovered an entirely new continent. Here he was at home. Schultz maintained that all the coffee he had previously drunk was mere dishwater, and he began his mission to bring this coffee experience to the American people (Schultz & Yang, 1997).

After having virtually begged to be allowed to work at Starbucks for one year, he was hired in 1982. He learned the art of coffee from the ground up, by working in the stores, speaking with those in the company who had a lot of knowledge and experience, tasting a lot of different kinds of coffee, and chatting with customers. Last, but not least, he learned how to roast coffee beans.

After one year, Schultz was sent to Milan, Italy, to take part in an international trade fair for housewares. On the very first day while wandering the streets of Milan, he discovered the espresso bars. There, for the first time, he witnessed the rituals and romance of the Italian espresso bars and saw how popular they were. The baristas, often wearing bow ties, knew just about everyone who stopped by and what kind of coffee they wanted. Opera music played continuously, and there were hardly any chairs in the premises because the espresso was consumed standing up. There was a pulsating energy as people congregated amidst the lovely aroma of roasted coffee beans. Schultz was enchanted. In the USA, there was nothing comparable and he brought these ideas home with him. Starbucks sold fantastic coffee beans, but they didn't sell ready-to-drink coffee by the cup. He believed recreating the authentic Italian coffee bar culture in the USA would give other Americans the chance to experience the same epiphany as Schultz had. Starbucks could become an experience, not just a store. This revelation was however not equally obvious to the owners of Starbucks. They didn't want to invest in a café enterprise and would not budge, regardless of how well Schultz formulated his arguments. This led to his forming his own company, Il Giornale. However, it didn't take long before the chance presented itself, and Schultz had the opportunity to take over Starbucks as CEO. The cafés that began under the name Il Giornale, were incorporated into Starbucks (Schultz & Yang, 1997).

When Il Giornale opened in 1986, it looked like the espresso bars Schultz had experienced in Milan, but is that what the Starbucks cafés are like today? No. The bow ties proved to be uncomfortable to work in. People complained about the endless opera music, and those who weren't in a hurry wanted to be able to sit down. Then there was the question of milk. Starbucks served only whole milk, because they believed that anything else would undermine the quality. Yes, the mere mention of low-fat milk was considered treason and led to the largest discussion in Starbucks's history. Schultz is purported to have said at one moment: "We will *never* serve low-fat milk! That's not who we are." Apparently, that's who they are now. Starbucks gradually evolved in response to its customers' feedback and wishes (Schultz & Yang, 1997).

When I started working in Stange, I made myself a promise. Before we started any services, programmes, or projects, we would always investigate whether this was actually something the population wanted. We would not tell people what we thought they needed, until we understood what they wanted.

Baby steps in Stange

In Stange, there were many factors in place to help build the kind of services I had been dreaming about. Fortunately, I wasn't alone in my ambitions. My superior, Liv Langberg, head of operations for children and family services in the municipality, had wanted to make this happen for several years. Liv is visionary, down to earth, generous, and clear, and she dares to go all out in her goals – everything I could have wished for from a leader. Liv often said, "We must start by setting goals. Then we can work backwards from there. In that way we will see what needs to be done." We had ambitions and monumental goals. Liv was always open to the possibility that the goals might have to be adjusted along the way and continually challenged us on how we envisioned the future. This type of flexibility in a leader is rare. Liv was also completely indispensable to Kårhild in terms of accomplishing what we wanted to do. In the organization, Kårhild worked upwards with grounding and downwards through involvement. He was constantly searching for external funding sources to support our efforts. We scoured the Norwegian Health Directorate's website on a regular basis in search of potential new resources we could apply to. When the state budget was announced, the relevant sections were printed and filed with opportunities marked for follow-up. Kårhild is thorough and has a formidable capacity to produce an overview, something which was wholly critical. If Stange had been a private company, Kårhild would have been the person who contacted countless potential sponsors to persuade them to invest in us. This was something else Howard Schultz had experienced at Starbucks. There wouldn't have been any Starbucks without the early investors.

For my own part I worked a lot on what the service should look like. We thought it was important to use ordinary language. If we were going to get people to talk with us, we had to speak a language that they understood. They had to recognize us as their equals, so they would be willing to share their thoughts and ideas with us. We wanted to make sure they would feel free to tell us what was important to them and what they thought was important in order for them to feel better and be well. What did they think would create change and growth in their lives? From there, we could in offer them our knowledge the next round, because one does not always personally know how to bring about the necessary changes in life. It's difficult to carry out such a job all alone, so people need someone to provide support along the way. Still, people know what is important to them and they have ideas about how they want to live their lives.

One of our first challenges was the name. We wanted a name that was simple and unassuming, a name the area residents might have come up with themselves. We did not want it filled with technical terms or words creating the aura of an organization. Trude Kjelgren from the mental health interest organization for children and young people (Mental Helse Ungdom) in Norway was included in our project group and we ran all the phrasing past her. "How does interdisciplinary team sound?" we asked. "No, that's too sinister," Trude said; "there's too much disciplinary-ness." So we dropped it. Sometimes Trude just said, "What are you actually talking about?" We then understood that we had to refine our approach. Previously we had had a small family team at the public health clinic, but now we wanted to avoid the word team. I told them about something called "The Helper" in Ski municipality, which I thought had a nice ring. It was one of the public health nurses who proposed "Family Help" (*Familiehjelpa*).

Plain and simple. It would later become Stangehelp, after the municipality in which we operate.

We started with almost nothing. My position was the only new addition in the municipality when we started up. But after an introductory tour through the other services in the municipality, we succeeded in convincing others that this was such a good idea that they would want to contribute from their own limited resources. We worked according to Petter Stordalen's strawberry philosophy. Stordalen (2009) is the owner and chairman of the board of Norway's largest hotel chain, Nordic Choice Hotels. He started his career at the age of 12, selling strawberries at the market in Porsgrunn. His father owned a grocery store and placed a small table and a mountain of strawberry crates in the middle of the square amidst all the market women. Petter had no chair, because his father believed he would sell less if he was seated. However, he knew that if he sold three crates very quickly then he could set the crates up on the ends and more or less rest his behind on them. The other strawberry salespeople had matching awnings, meticulously handwritten signs, and overflowing baskets. One evening in the car when Petter and his father were on their way to pick up another load of berries, he fretted to his father: "I want better berries, a cooler parasol, maybe bigger table?" Then his father said: "Sell the berries you have, because they are the only berries you can sell. It doesn't help to complain about everything you don't have. If you are going to accomplish something, start with what you have!" That night, before he fell asleep, Petter thought: "My father is a genius!" He stands by that to this day.

Although Kårhild was constantly searching for state funding, we knew that we needed help from the other services within the municipality. We had to use what we already had to get things rolling. Both the child welfare service and the public health clinic took part and contributed resources. Eventually we had found enough people to enable us to start operation of Stangehelp. There weren't many of us, and we didn't want to spread ourselves too thin, so we decided to limit the service to families with children aged 0–6 years. We had made up our minds to provide services that would enable us to show results at an early stage and simultaneously acquire such a good reputation in the municipality that they wouldn't want to do without us. Instead of creating something that was a bit half-baked for many people, our goal was to produce the very best service for families with preschool-age children. We painstakingly recorded the results of the work and communicated this to the municipal management, politicians, and everyone willing to listen to us. We believed that an expansion would take time, but two successful applications for extra resources from state funding were granted, which made it possible to expand the service offer to include all the children in the municipality and their families. However, because these resources were only for a limited duration, for a short time we were afraid we would have to phase out the service for schoolchildren. Fortunately, the political leadership of the municipality thought differently and ensured that funds were included in the budget to secure the programme. Stangehelp was saved. Throughout this entire process, the most important concerns were results and our reputation within the population. We were at the beginning of what seemed a great adventure. What would come to secure our existence and continued development was our commitment to the residents that we would be the best mental health care service for the individual and, in the long term, the best mental health care service for the municipality as a whole. If we had not focused on this, we would certainly never have managed to develop the service so successfully. At the end of 2013, all six of the other services in the municipality contributed resources to Stangehelp, which demonstrated that people thought we were a worthwhile investment.

There are many advantages to taking small steps when you are going to create something new. In his book *Little Bets: How Breakthrough Ideas Emerge from Small Discoveries*, author Peter Sims (2011) makes the argument that truly innovative companies don't start with big ideas. They discover them along the way. He maintains that one should embrace the uncertainty and be willing to experiment, working through trial and error, but do so on such a small scale that occasional missteps don't matter. Some efforts won't lead to anything big, but now and then a new idea or procedure can yield fantastic results. True innovators don't analyse new ideas too much, or make plans that are so big that they stake everything on one strategy. Neither do they carry out precise analyses in advance of what they believe the outcome will be. Instead they learn *by doing something to discover what they should do.* They build stone by stone and can therefore make whatever adjustments become necessary along the way without losing too much. Learning is viewed in the same way that many others view failure: by making small mistakes quickly, we learn more in a shorter time period and can in the long run invest resources with far greater expedience. Small successes offer wholly different opportunities to acquire further resources, because these are based on success. This doesn't mean that we should throw all caution to the wind. The most productive, creative innovators are thorough, extremely analytical, strategic, and pragmatic.

Within the public sector unfortunately very little is done in this way. Instead, huge reforms are implemented and virtually impossible to evaluate. If something doesn't produce results, it is considered a failure, and the politicians who initiated the reform are driven to the wall. Because they are concerned about justifying their decisions, they will seek to wiggle their way out of the accusations, fight back, or otherwise seek to maintain their position. It becomes important to minimize the risk of making a mistake, and an experimental approach becomes impossible. There has been investment in such types of reforms in the public sector of Norway for many years, within the school system, the public health sector, and other areas of public administration. When systems don't function as intended, it is often believed that the solution lies in either spending more money or reorganizing. Quality has also become a popular buzzword in all contexts. "Quality enhancement" in the schools, "quality indicators" within the health care sector, and "quality reforms" and "quality assurance" take on paramount importance. The contents are presumed to be different, but that is seldom the case. It also becomes very difficult to know what has been good and what has been less good about a reform, because at best only isolated parts of it are evaluated. Only rarely is a programme revoked after it has been implemented. After a "new" measure entails a large upheaval and economic investment, an evaluation which could demonstrate that it was a mistake is virtually impossible. In such cases, it is not careful, deliberate steps that lead reform; instead there has been a large investment in an idea that is produced far away from the grass roots. This is a paradox when we know that it is precisely from grass roots that the best ideas come.

To ensure quality, control mechanisms are also implemented and reported on by the public sector to the central public authorities in the form of quantifiable results. This could at best be viewed as a kind of feedback which could be applied to make improvements. The problem is that most reporting systems aren't suited as a medium for learning, because what is being reported on doesn't correspond with the service's own priorities. When anticipating and learning from mistakes are not a part of the mentality, the reporting becomes more a mechanism that produces fear and inhibits creativity and development.

A substantial adjustment of the attitude in programme management has been necessary in order to achieve truly good results; this can often be the case in programmes around the world. Stangehelp has been fortunate enough to have escaped the politics that hinder our ability to create something new within mental health care. This doesn't mean that we can do whatever we want. We submit regular reports on what we are doing, how we are doing it, and the results we have achieved in the form of simple statistics. The difference is that we do this because we believe it is important in order for us to learn something and for us to recognize which path we must follow. The reporting is not used as a control mechanism, but as feedback for ourselves. Because we take baby steps at all times, we can try things out that we don't absolutely know will work, without it mattering very much if we fail now and then. The best ideas come from the field, and they come gradually. Making large-scale plans at a level far removed from where the services are provided will usually lead to poorer quality. At the same time, it becomes difficult to make changes along the way. Baby steps, based on local ideas and hands-on world experience of what works, can offer a lot of insight and learning, using minimal resources and in a short period of time. As Thomas Edison said, "If I find 10,000 ways something won't work, I haven't failed. I am not discouraged, because every wrong attempt discarded is often a step forward."

The operation of Stangehelp was founded on the principles of deliberate practice explained in Chapter 4. There are few guidelines available for how this can be done in organizations, so we had to find inspiration from many sources. Our work is based on Ericsson's research on expertise, but it has been equally important to derive inspiration from literature about companies and organizations that have succeeded. Understanding what the companies that really succeed have done helped us to sort out where we must focus and what is not as important.

The development of outstanding individual therapists is not enough in the long run. We must become proficient together. Only then can our efforts produce ripple effects in society.

This is how your organization will become one of the best

Define your market

Throughout most of the 19th and 20th centuries the railway was the most successful industry in the USA. Different companies competed on laying track from city to city throughout the continent, increasing the speed and earning a lot of money in the process. However, in the 1960s this once-vital stakeholder in American commerce experienced a serious, almost fatal, downturn. When people went looking for explanations, the general opinion was that the need was met by others (such as automobiles, trucks, aeroplanes, and new technology such as the telephone). It was difficult to refute such arguments. When it came to transport, consumers wanted faster, simpler, and more individualized solutions. Harvard professor Theodore Levitt questioned this logic. He said that the railway industry had problems "not because the need was met by others but because it was not met by the railroad companies themselves". Why didn't the railway industry evolve when it had the chance? This may have been because the railway directors believed they were in the railway business rather than in the transportation business (Levitt, 1960). Thus, trucking and airline industries flourished while the old iron horse rusted away.

As we develop services within mental health, we must know what business we are working in. The way we define our industry will be critical to the way we learn and improve ourselves or, as blogger and author Cal Newport put it, our success in the marketplace within which we are operating. For a long time, Newport was interested in understanding how certain people become very good at something. After completing his doctorate at the Massachusetts Institute of Technology and before he was hired by the Department of Computer Science at Georgetown University, he wrote the book *So Good They Can't Ignore You* (Newport, 2012). In the book he tries to understand how some people become very good at what they do, while at the same time they do it with enthusiasm and love. Part of this is about the market. If you are going to become very good at, for example, playing the violin, running marathons, or writing a novel, you need to become very good at specific skills, and that is all that matters. If you practise this in a goal-oriented, deliberate fashion, you will probably succeed. Newport calls this a "winner-takes-all-market". If, on the other hand, you work with developmental aid or environmental issues, for example, the market is much less structured, and you need different types of knowledge. Newport calls this an "auction market".

The problem with the mental health care field is that we often seem to believe we are in a winner-takes-all-market. If we become very good at psychotherapy, then we will succeed. However, we are actually an auction market, because there are so very many different things that produce change in people. Bruce Wampold, mentioned in Chapter 2, has been saying this for more than 10 years. When people who do therapy change, only 13% of this change can be attributed to the treatment effect, while 87% can be attributed to everything else (also referred to as extra-therapeutic/client factors). So, while we are busy figuring out the next miracle method, we are missing the mark on 87% of the market. Perhaps it's not so strange that the field is stagnating?

Care about results

The employees of LEGO were deeply invested in LEGO. Their pride in the product they created meant they could not imagine working anywhere else. They wore t-shirts bearing the slogan "Only the best is good enough", not because they had to but because they believed it. CEO Knudstorp believes this might be one of the reasons things started to go wrong. The company had never operated with a loss before 1998, and a sense of complacency had set in. Profits and money were not discussed; they were viewed as something negative that clashed with the company's culture. The LEGO founder, Ole Kirk Christiansen, viewed LEGO more as a standard for high-quality toys that stimulated learning and creativity than as a commercial product. This had always been LEGO's teaching, but at the beginning of the new millennium this philosophy began leading the company towards bankruptcy. Owing to a large drop in sales and increase in debt, LEGO was obliged to adapt. For the employees it meant that, instead of losing themselves in the subtleties of product development, they had to recognize the company's bottom line as their primary concern. Salaries were based partly on performance, and employees were expected to work more quickly. Where previously the development of an idea into a finished product had taken two years, it now took 12 months. In order for the company to survive, results rather than employees' preferences would have to determine their future course. Their increased efficiency contributed to greater effectiveness (Robertson & Breen, 2013).

Effectiveness is a difficult word in the mental health field. Often when I have spoken about this to other therapists or managers, they wrinkle their brows and their entire face tells me this is a word they don't like. Some state explicitly that this is a negative word for them, and they don't think it should enter the process. In part, this is about a misunderstanding of the meaning of the word. Some people believe that effectiveness is about doing something very quickly. Within the field of mental health care, that means we are supposed to practise a form of short-term therapy that is completed quickly. This contradicts a fundamental attitude within the field that change requires time. However, effectiveness is not necessarily about something happening quickly. Effectiveness is about added value and the wise use of resources. True effectiveness means achieving high valued added goals while using fewer resources. Essentially, the outcome is worth more than the resources used to achieve it. Effectiveness is more than just productivity, which is about the volume of production relative to the use of resources.

First and foremost, high level of value creation produces good results for consumers of the service. This means that they experience improvement or achieve something they personally view as being valuable, and thus resources are devoted to meet consumer needs. Value creation in terms of human services can be about enhanced quality of life, fewer symptoms, job performance mastery, or social relationships. Essentially, it means fostering an experience of greater satisfaction with oneself and others. Only those we are going to help are in a position to know where they want to be, what they need help with, and whether their goals and needs are being met, so we must listen to them. The feedback tool described in Chapter 3 is a valuable mechanism for collecting this kind of information.

At Stangehelp, we have focused on results from the very beginning. In this way, we established the basis to justify continuing our work. We showed our results to political leaders, and they agreed that the municipality should continue to support our work. In order to communicate with the local community about what we were doing, and with an eye towards our own development, we started mapping out everything we did at an early stage. We sat down and decided what kind of systematic knowledge we would need to keep track of, including the reasons why people contacted us, the type of help they wanted, how long we had contact with them, and factors in their lives that created difficulties for them. Next, we created categories within the respective areas, based not on our own preconceived notions but rather on what the families themselves told us. These categories were not defined until after we had been working on the system for a while, and they undergo continual adjustment. Our statistics therefore change a little each year, in accordance with what is important for the families. We also use Feedback-Informed Treatment (FIT) on all the families in order to gain an overview of how many clients experience improvement while they are in contact with us and how they experience the time spent with us. All this information helps us determine where we must make improvements, particularly where we need additional expertise. The information also helps us to set goals for the service and to know what we should strive for in the way of results, in keeping with what the respective families experience as being important in their lives.

Good outcomes for individuals or families are important, but equally important are the results affecting the local community. A mental health care service should be concerned with results that have an impact beyond the identified client's personal circumstances. Is there a decline in the incidence of mental health disorders in the community? Is there a reduction in the number of people on sick leave or disability due to mental health disorders? Is there a decrease in the number of high school dropouts? Do the child welfare services receive fewer reports of concern? How many people commit suicide? How many children are bullied at school? Community mental health care providers should be interested in such results to a much greater extent and collaborate with other services towards a common goal. That means we must expand our reach. This will also enable us to bring about advancement in the field.

Start developing the culture right away

Early in the development of Stangehelp, we began working with culture and values. We'd read Ingebrigt Steen Jensen's (2002) book *One Lighthouse* (*Ona fyr*), which helped us to understand that to succeed we had to develop a common understanding – "this is how we work here". We held in-house seminars where brainstorming sessions and Post-its abounded. Finally, we settled on three basic values: down to earth, flexible, and helpful. We also worked on formulating a vision for the service, which turned out to be an arduous affair. After one year of back and forth, we ended up with the following:

Stange municipality will be a good municipality to live in.

- We believe in people's potential.
- We want to help families help themselves.
- We will be humble, listen, and dare to try out unfamiliar strategies.
- It is the people we help who determine whether we succeed.

Our values and vision help us make decisions about where to invest our efforts. We can test many things, but if something contradicts our values, we drop it right away. Our values play a part in creating the culture of the service. A lot has been written about organizational culture, but you don't actually need to be an expert to achieve this. The culture grows out of working towards the same goal and being faithful to the values. It is difficult to change an established culture. If one has been working in a certain way for many years, a new set of values will be experienced more as a disturbance. In starting a new service, one must communicate the values up front and let them serve as guidelines for everything, from the hiring of new employees to the development of the service offer. For managers and employees alike, the most important thing is to communicate the values to one another and especially to new employees. Not much more than this is required.

In addition to our values, there is a clear expectation that we will achieve high-level performance. We must be the best service for the families who come into contact with us. Developing a culture that emphasizes performance excellence is not always easy, especially if in an already-established "good enough" culture. The employees will not automatically embrace such a change. Robbie Babins-Wagner, chief executive officer of Calgary Counseling Centre, has 62 employees who meet 8,000 new clients each year. In 2000, she started establishing a culture that made performance excellence a top priority and this remains an ongoing process. As she expected, this was a very difficult process. Initially, she experienced a staff turnover rate of as much as 40%. Babins-Wagner emphasizes that changing the way one works in a large organization will inevitably involve a certain amount of negativity and dismissals (Babins-Wagner, 2017).

Invest in your leaders

> Leadership is communicating to people their worth and potential so clearly that they are inspired to see it in themselves.
>
> Stephen R. Covey

We can divide leaders into roughly two types: those who are good at administration and those who are good at leading (and then, of course, there are those who are good at both or neither). Leaders who are just good at administration are not really leaders. They are managers. They keep the shop running smoothly, watch the bottom line, make sure employees receive what they're entitled to, and assure the organization complies with pertinent laws and regulations – but they don't lead. A true leader has a vision for the organization, a deeper idea about why it exists and a clear perception of where it should be headed. The leader has a standard for how the company should perform, speaks about the vision in every context, and represents what the company wants to achieve. In the mental health care service, unfortunately, we have far too many managers. They work hard to fulfil the requirements of top management and the public authorities, count what needs to be counted, and make as few waves as possible. However, what we need are leaders who can take the field of mental health care to new levels, leaders who have ambitions to develop the profession, to do things in new ways, to challenge existing practice, and to improve results by thinking innovatively. This requires courage.

Developing good leaders should be an integrated and given aspect of the mental health care services. Good leadership is not about the type of professional training one has. Good psychologists can be good leaders or terrible leaders. This holds true for physicians, nurses, or any other occupational group. Identifying and developing promising leaders early on gives the organization enormous advantages, but cultivating leaders is not a job to be taken lightly. By challenging employees and allowing them to try out different leadership tasks, one can give them opportunities to become leaders. Leadership is a large, specialized field, and a lot has been written about what makes somebody a good leader. I will limit myself to a few characteristics that I have taken from *One Lighthouse* (Jensen, 2002) and which are important elements of the deliberate practice mindset.

- The leader must have an understanding that his or her most important task is to contribute to pursuing the vision established for the company. This person must have an ambition of steering the company towards a constant desire to improve and reach the objectives it has set.
- The leader must have the humility required to disclose his or her own limitations and be able to admit when he or she is wrong. The leader must be able to make a lot of concessions, but *never give an inch* on the core contents of the vision.
- The leader must stand behind what the service represents, even in times of turbulence or when this makes him or her unpopular. The leader must be driven enough to accept the consequences of their choices that have been made and to implement decisions.
- The leader must have an ability to put together a team that includes some who are good at something and others at something else, because diversity promotes development. The leader must also have the wisdom to allow all the employees create, own, and take responsibility for the objectives the department has set.

Ingebrigt Steen Jensen summarizes this nicely in his book (2002):

> Bad leaders are bad at sharing, whether it's a matter of knowledge, power or money. And they are unsurpassed when it comes to saying no and but. "No," they say, "we can't do this because we've never done it before." And if that doesn't do the trick, they say "No, we

> can't do this because we *have* done it before." The best leaders are the exact opposite. They say no if they must and then because the idea does not correspond with the vision, value base, objectives and journey. But they say yes if they can. They listen if people have something to say, they sparkle if somebody turns on the light, celebrate if there is something good on the horizon.
>
> (Jensen, 2002)

This is how you develop your team

A good leader must be able to share. Oversized egos have no place in good leadership. Good leadership is about joining together with others and hiring people with knowledge or abilities you may lack. Leaders may not possess all the good characteristics all by themselves. They need to be surrounded by people who will complement their skills and step in when the leader needs a break. One feature of the truly successful companies is that they were started by more than one person. There is always a "we" rather than an "I". Liv, Kårhild, and I worked as a team of three at the start, along with all the others in the municipality who contributed to the development of Stangehelp. Over time, I realized that I needed somebody with whom I could share responsibility for daily operations. I needed somebody who shared the vision and values of Stangehelp but who was also smart, creative, and able to offer own ideas for development. Leaders who surround themselves exclusively with devoted helpmates will find it difficult to grow as an organization. Any successful team requires strong, secure individuals who are not afraid to speak up when they disagree and fight for their own ideas while remaining faithful to the core values of the organization.

Bjørnar Fauske Bye was recruited to Stangehelp when we were going to expand in 2012. I needed somebody who could step in for me and be responsible for the work targeting schoolchildren. Bjørnar had previously been employed at the Hagen treatment centre, so I knew he already had the right values. Simultaneously, he was different enough from me that he would bring something new into the service. When I run out of ideas for improvement, Bjørnar suggests something unexpected that I have not considered. Most important: Bjørnar can keep up with Stangehelp's steep learning curve, which comes with always asking for feedback from the families.

With strong leaders, it's possible to get to work on developing the team. The staff constitutes an organization's most valuable asset. If the staff doesn't function, neither will the organization. Excellent services come from the combined efforts of individual employees. Taking care of the staff is, therefore, one of a leader's most important tasks. Staff must feel valued, significant, and able to identify with the vision of the service so they experience ownership in relation between established goals and end results.

Mental health care services exist in an auction market. That means we need employees with different combinations of skills, and these must be developed in accordance with the requirements of market demand. Each individual employee must be developed, and it is crucial to be aware of how they complement one another. When hiring new staff, it's vital to identify the required skills or qualities and communicate this clearly in the hiring process. That is what we did with Marie.

We hired Marie Klæt Gjersheim in the autumn of 2012. She was a recent psychology graduate and one of many applicants who wanted to become a part of Stangehelp. The applicants included recent graduates, others with some experience, and a number of specialists. Marie stood out at the interview. She had an enormous desire to learn; in truth, she seemed to love learning. She was fond of reading and asked if we had any suggestions for books she could read during her summer vacation before starting to work for us. As a recent graduate she understood that she did not have all the answers, but she wanted a role in the process of our gradually developing our service and finding out what would be helpful to our clients.

When asked to tell us what is important for her with an eye to her development and improvement of her skills, Marie says loudly and clearly: "Supervision!". Marie finds it helpful to receive suggestions and advice on what she can do differently if she should get stuck. She admits that she doesn't always know what to do and may need help to work out alternative courses of action. For her it is important that her supervisor be clear and honest and give her something concrete to work with. She also wants reading suggestions and makes it a priority to make time for reading. Marie uses her supervision to develop her knowledge base. Like a chess player, she wants to have as many moves at her disposal as possible when she is sitting with a family or a child. By having constant access to feedback, Marie can always cultivate her knowledge and adjust her approach as needed. She doesn't waste her own time or the time of the family by insisting that they work according to her rules if it does not help them.

Identifying promising employees at an early stage and starting to cultivate them gives an organization many advantages. You capitalize on each individual staff member's full potential and need not wait until they have completed certain courses or acquired sufficient seniority. Giving employees tasks that challenge them from the very start helps to identify areas in which the individual will flourish. We all have different ambitions and preferences for how we want to work. At the same time, it is important to challenge the employees to step out of their comfort zone, where they can discover tasks that previously seemed beyond the scope of their abilities, now become exciting.

The best organizations cultivate their employees in much the same manner as coaches within sports or music teachers who choose exercises for their students: by pushing them a bit beyond their abilities and challenging them to learn new skills. The most effective way of encouraging people to extend themselves is by assigning tasks outside their comfort zones. This sounds simple, but can be complicated. Many organizations have a tendency to give people tasks that fit the areas in which they already excel rather than those in which they need to develop their skills. In the short term, this can seem like the best solution because the ongoing work requirement would recommend the best prepared individuals for specific tasks. In the long term, however, this leads to less growth and development for the overall organization, because the individual employee's development comes to a halt.

Expanding the skills of all employees will not only bring good results for your organization; it will also create an appealing workplace that will attract more qualified people. Ultimately, there will be less fear of losing qualified professionals in whose development the organization has invested time and resources. There will always be new candidates to fill expanding roles, and those who need new challenges in other places in order to develop will have the opportunity to pursue them.

What motivates excellent performance

In order for employees to excel at their jobs, they need motivation. A good deal of research has explored what motivates us to solve demanding tasks. We must bring the findings of this type of research into the organization. In his TED talk and book *Drive: the Surprising Truth about What Motivates Us*, Daniel H. Pink (2009) has demonstrated that there is a considerable discrepancy between what research tells us about motivation and what companies actually do.

Pink starts by describing what he calls the Motivation 2.0 system (Motivation 1.0 consisted of our basic drives). This type of motivation is predominantly about achieving a reward or avoiding punishment. Motivation 2.0 has existed within working life for a long time and has functioned well in many ways; otherwise it would hardly have survived for such a long time. During the industrial revolution, workers were viewed as parts of a complex machine. The objective was to get them to do their parts of the job in the right way at the right time so the machine would run smoothly. In order to ensure this, leaders would reward desirable behaviour and sanction undesirable behaviour. Employees would respond to this rationally, and both they and the system would benefit from such an approach. This type of approach to motivation is often called "the carrot and stick approach". In other words, it is based on motivational factors that are external.

The problem with such an approach is that it does not function as well on complicated tasks in which new, more flexible solutions must be applied. Thus, Motivation 2.0 has run into some resistance in recent times. In 2002, Nobel laureate Daniel Kahneman caused us to think differently about what we do and questioned many of the assumptions underlying Motivation 2.0. Specifically, he suggested that human beings are much more irrational than we believe. The underlying assumptions of Motivation 2.0 hold that we are rational, robot-like producers who will always respond correctly to the carrot and the stick. Sometimes we do, but usually we don't. Why doesn't such an approach to motivation work? It can be a source of incitement for cheating and make us narrow-minded in our way of thinking. It can also make tasks seem less interesting than they need to be, while creativity and performance excellence receive a cold shower (Kahneman, 2011).

What we need is a full-scale upgrade of our motivation system. If one is going to move a pile of sand from one place to another using a shovel, reward is a fine type of motivation. However, in most knowledge-driven jobs, this works poorly. Motivation 3.0, on the other hand, relies more on inner motivation. This type of motivation is less concerned with the reward and more with the inner satisfaction of a job well done.

Motivation 3.0 is made up of three elements. The first is *autonomy*. A clear example of this is something called results-only work environment (ROWE), which has been implemented by some companies. This is a radical means of giving employees autonomy in their own work. There are no office hours. One need not turn up at a specific place at a specific time. How they do their jobs, when they do them, and where they do them is up to the employees. The only thing that matters is that they get the job done. This approach is not possible in all services. Some workplaces require workers to be present because the work involves helping other people. Still, there is something valuable about this kind of mindset. The public sector of Norway uses some form of time cards on a broad scale. In other words, it's not that important whether or not the job gets done as long as the employee can document that they were at work for a sufficient number of hours every day. Giving employees autonomy is about arranging the working conditions so the they can do the best possible job. Instead of trying to control employees, leaders are supposed to awaken their inner need for autonomy. At first, the transition to such a mentality can be difficult; the employees are not accustomed to it and it can be perceived as unsafe. However, if the organization succeeds in introducing a culture in which autonomy is valued, this will lead to more creativity and give the employees the security to try out new ideas. In the long term, this can produce far better performances than a more controlled environment. Some people believe that trying out new ideas, and perhaps making mistakes with some of them, is an expensive way of running a service, but in the long run it is cheaper. Mediocrity is expensive, and mediocrity stems from control and rigid routines.

The second element is *mastery*. Mastery means gaining competence or improving skills at what one does and producing results. One of the employees of Stangehelp said once, "You know, Birgit, even though we work in a municipal service, we still want to improve and see results from what we are doing." This says something about the culture and attitudes towards performance within the public sector of Norway. Controlling routines lead to people conforming to the system, while autonomy leads to engagement. Only engagement can produce truly high-level performance. Employees work better in conditions that facilitate mastery and outcome visibility. This engenders commitment and improved performance.

The last element is *meaning*. The most motivated people are those who appreciate that they are working for something that is larger than themselves. I have asked the employees of Stangehelp about what motivates them to work the way we do, with high performance requirements and an expectation that the individual will continually be developing and improving both their own and the service's performance. One of the employees said, "It is because I believe in this."

The public sector of Norway faces a number of challenges with respect to the motivation of employees. Since the 1990s, Norwegian public administration has been reformed in the direction of what is called new public management. This ideology includes both market mechanisms and control routines. New reporting systems are introduced all the time, something that allegedly assures the quality of the individual service. The mountains of forms and required report writing have increased to such an extent that many employees spend substantially more time on this than on their actual jobs, i.e. providing services for the population. Upward loyalty is important in such a system. Employees are expected to carry out assignments determined by the level above, while that level is loyal to the level above it in turn. It is important to avoid making mistakes and to minimize risk, so no grit arises that will prevent the machine from running smoothly. Any mistake would make the leaders look bad, which in turn would have an impact on the politicians who have passed the reforms derived from this management system. Control routines can lead to the fear of making mistakes on the part of employees. In the worst-case scenario, they may refrain from doing anything at all.

Many public sectors need adjustment in their management ideology. Developing a service in accordance with deliberate practice becomes virtually impossible within a system that shuns mistakes and deprives employees of autonomy. The public services can provide ample opportunity to ensure that employees can experience an exceptionally high level of *meaning* in their work. Most of what we do is about helping others and creating a better society, but this intention is drowned in bureaucracy and compulsory tasks that are meaningless. When you can't see the results of what you do, you will eventually stop caring about what you do and you will not improve.

The road ahead

The field of mental health care is like the very first Starbucks café. There are no chairs in the room. The opera music grates in people's ears, and the bow ties get in the way of performance excellence. Besides, people want something besides whole milk. They want low-fat milk. Yes, they might even want soy milk.

If we invest the time and effort to listen to people, we will begin to see unimagined possibilities. We will begin to discern the contours of where this field can go. We can make large discoveries, receive some uncomfortable surprises, and be astonished at how simple the complex can be – and how complicated something simple can be. At Stangehelp, we experience this every day. The next chapter offers responses from some of those we have asked. What do those we are actually supposed to help tell us about what is important to them? What do we have to learn?

7

LISTEN!

Most people do not listen with the intent to understand; they listen with the intent to reply.

Stephen R. Covey

In the early 1970s, Ernesto Sirolli worked for an Italian organization that provided developmental aid in Africa. The organization was interested in promoting the development of trade and industry and sent out volunteers to implement projects in collaboration with the local residents of the relevant nations. Sirolli was hired by the organization to monitor the volunteers, which brought him to Chirundu, a village in Zambia near the Zambezi River. The developmental plan for the village included that 30 men would work every day to prepare the soil for the cultivation of tomatoes and other vegetables. The men would eventually assume responsibility for the land and be allowed to use all the resources the Italians had brought with them – a tractor, trucks, storage facilities, seeds, and other equipment. On the whole, it appeared to be a good plan, but before long problems arose. The men came to work on the first Monday, but then they didn't come back again, at least not for the next six days (Sirolli, 1999).

The Italians eventually understood that a kwacha (which at the time was worth about one US dollar), which the employees received for one day's work, was enough money to buy sufficient corn flour for a whole week. Corn flour was the main staple of the village diet and had to be bought, while they could get fish from the river and game from the forest. Quite simply, the men did not need to work more than one day in order to feed their families with what they needed for an entire week.

When the Italians realized this, they despaired. What about their results? How would they meet the obligations they had in relation to the Italian and Zambian governments if the men would only work on Mondays? They couldn't reduce their salaries, because the agreement with the Zambian government was a minimum wage of one kwacha per day. What should they do? The Italian volunteers came up with an original solution to an unusual problem. They induced the local men to want more money by encouraging them to buy goods that the Italians owned, such as sunglasses, watches, radios, beer, and whisky. In the course of six months they had conquered Chirundu (Sirolli, 1999).

Now the men worked every day, except for a few of them who failed to turn up on Monday because they were hungover. Sirolli was incredulous about what had happened. Here they were supposed to be helping these people, but instead they had made them dependent on beer so that they would want more money, and therefore come to work. At the time, Sirolli was too young to object and too naive not to believe their arguments about how it was the results that mattered. He therefore said nothing, convinced that if he had been one of the volunteers he would have done the same thing. He would have "motivated" the local men, found a way to make the project "a success" and "achieve the goals" that had been set. However, that was before Sirolli saw the results of the tomato farming (Sirolli, 1999).

The tomato seeds that had been shipped from Italy had thrived particularly well in the fertile African soil by the bank of the Zambezi River. They had grown into gigantic plants that were a sight to behold against the blue water. Unfortunately, one morning when the time came to harvest the crop, the Italian volunteers had gone to the field and found nothing but large pools of water where the plants had been. Nothing was left. It looked as if somebody had dug the plants up in a completely haphazard manner. It didn't take long to figure out what had happened; all one had to do was to follow the ripples on the water. A herd of hippopotamuses were taking siesta just a stone's throw away, well-fed on what had been the pride and joy of the Italians' development aid work (Sirolli, 1999).

The Italians were upset and went to the local men to tell them what had happened. The men, however, took the news with a stunning complacency and simply replied, "This is the reason we don't have agriculture in Zambia." The Italians looked at them in astonishment and asked, "But why didn't you tell us?" The men replied, "You never asked" (Sirolli, 1999).

Sirolli's experiences from Africa in the 1970s have shaped everything he has done since. He became convinced that what they did in Africa was not right and that very much of what they did actually created more problems than it solved. In 1973, E.F. Schumacher's book *Small Is Beautiful* offered some revolutionary ideas that challenged the experts' established truths about what brings about development. The book taught Sirolli two things: first, if people don't ask for help, leave them alone. Second, there is no good or bad way to carry out a task; there are only suitable or unsuitable ways. Figuring out which is suitable depends completely upon the circumstances. Schumacher emphasized that one shouldn't assume that it's possible to identify other people's problems and provide solutions that are correct for the situation in question. One must have respect for the experiences of others, wait until one is invited to share their problems, listen with an open mind, and abandon one's own prejudices and any assumptions that one knows best. Schumacher was an economist and spoke about the economy, but this wasn't strictly about economics. Sirolli immediately knew that the focus had to be on human beings, that they were what mattered. Schumacher concludes his book with these words:

> Everywhere people ask: "What can I actually do?" The answer is as simple as it is disconcerting; we can each of us, put our inner house in order. The guidance we need for this work cannot be found in

science or technology, the value of which utterly depends on the ends they serve; but it can still be found in the traditional wisdom of mankind.

After this lesson, Sirolli's work took another direction. He became interested in human development and read everything he could about the subject. This led him to the work of Abraham Maslow (1968). What did one need to put one's "inner house in order"? Maslow was fascinated by the wise, psychologically healthy people he had met, and he studied them. From here, he developed his pyramid of needs through which he held could tell us in which direction we needed to move in order to grow. Maslow maintained that there are no limits to personal growth and that an inherent human characteristic is a constant desire to fulfil one's needs. He claimed that, once our physiological needs, such as hunger and sleep, are met, our needs become psychological. In other words, when we are no longer hungry or tired, we are not actually interested in acquiring even more things. Instead, we become interested in whom we can become. Security is the first non-physiological need, and when this is met we experience a desire for love, group belonging, and social acceptance. For a secure and loved person, respect and self-respect will be important. At the top if the pyramid, however, is what Maslow calls self-realization.

Sirolli understood that development was a never-ending process and that it was more about psychological needs than material needs. Successful development was dependent upon quality not quantity. Sirolli began the task of finding out what type of service was needed to maximize the number of people who could grow to their full potential. If healthy people created healthy societies, they should then be concerned about creating structures that promote personal growth. Sirolli was profoundly inspired by Carl Rogers and the way he communicated with people to support their growth and development. It was the individual who was central, not the problem, and the goal was to foster person grow rather than solve a specific problem. Rogers' therapy was not about changing the individual but about removing hindrances to personal growth. Rogers could see people's hidden potential, the fulfilment of which required only that their needs for love and respect be met.

Sirolli brought these ideas with him in his work on developing local communities all over the world. By removing barriers adults can manage their own lives, take care of their children, work, and give back to society in a positive way. Sirolli is not a psychologist or a therapist, but his book, *Ripples from the Zambezi* (Sirolli, 1999), is a brilliant example of how to go about creating change in people, which has consequences for the larger society.

Sirolli's message is this: If you are going to help somebody, you must believe in them. Individuals are valuable; they can improve themselves, create value, and become better human beings. You must be good at communicating, but the most important thing is not saying magic words to a client. Instead, be a good listener. With adequate prompting and support, people will open up and share their innermost thoughts. In therapy, we must help people help themselves. The beginning of communication is about being passive. This can seem odd in our action-oriented culture, which has little comprehension for the value of being passive. However, by being passive, the relationship between client and helper is reversed: it is the client who is in control. If we start doing things right away, people begin to view us as experts. Then they will also begin to doubt their everyday ideas. Experts represent authority, and authority can be frightening. This will not promote the client's growth and development, but inhibit it instead.

When a therapist has heard their clients' own ideas, they can start to work. Then as a helper, a therapist can listen to the client and his or her ideas, make suggestions and share knowledge about what is required to achieve what the client wants. However, the therapist should never take over the project, never takes control of some aspects of another person's life. It is predominantly a matter of an attitude. Things happen because we believe in people, because we are positive and earnest in our work and desire to see others succeed.

If you want to help somebody, shut up and listen!

When I saw Sirolli's TED Talk, titled "If you want to help someone, shut up and listen!", for the first time, I was captivated. I watched it over and over again and thought long and hard about how his principles could be transferred to the field of mental health care. He spoke about so many of the things that we had just begun to develop at Stangehelp, and he confirmed ideas we had barely dared to consider. Was this really possible? Could the users be seated in the driver's seat as we advanced the field of mental health care? Are their ideas better than ours? Would ideas from the grass-roots level, from people themselves, be better than those coming from experts, professional expertise, and research communities? Is that where the potential for development lies, that which will move the field forward?

Sirolli bases his work on psychological theories about growth and development. The idea is that if individuals are happy and doing well in a society, they will produce values and contribute to a better, richer, and more enlightened society. It is *human beings* who cause a country to flourish, and their dreams are important. The fundamental belief in human nature – the belief that people can grow to full maturity and become good human beings – is what drives Sirolli. His ideas can offer insight to the field of mental health care. The development of therapy models has focused more on experts defining methods and making all the rules. Trained experts can assume that the people we meet in the field of mental health care are too sick, too disturbed for a truly collaborative approach. They need our expert help, somebody who can tell them what they need to do to get well. Had they had these answers themselves, certainly they wouldn't have found themselves in such a difficult situation.

I contacted Sirolli to discuss these questions. He wrote back, explaining that many doctors think that there are healthy people and there are sick people. He and his group, on the other hand, believe that each of us is situated somewhere on a continuum between "a vegetative state and the enlightened saint". All humans face challenges and have opportunities. He said that clients experiencing many challenges have extremely modest needs compared with those who have great ambitions. However, for them the realization of some small dreams will give them enormous personal satisfaction, and that is enough. His clients tell him that having contact with one of his helpers gave permission to dream again. When a person experiencing great challenges experiences success, this becomes an example to be followed by the rest of the local society. If he/she could do it, so can I!

Sirolli didn't need feedback scales when he was sitting at the café on the corner and making himself available to listen to people's ideas, but neither did he work within a system designed with a strong emphasis on the importance of expert competence and a predominant tendency to take effective action. As experts, we are eager to do something, and when we become very active there is a risk that those we are supposed to be helping will become passive. In his book, Sirolli (1999) suggests that the person who is a hurry to start doing things immediately quickly gets identified as an expert – a person who will develop others. From there, those in need of help become spectators who merely watch while the expert does things for them. Thus, it becomes difficult for them to confide in the expert, precisely because they are an expert and presumably know best. Nonetheless, our clients try to give us feedback all the time, sometimes implicitly and quietly, while other feedback is virtually shouted at us. It is up to us to receive the feedback and act accordingly. Do we dare take in the most obvious feedback? The following offers some examples of this.

The obvious forms of feedback

On 22 August 2013, I sat in the auditorium of the Fritt Ord Foundation on Parkveien in Oslo. It was my first time attending Amalie Days, an annual mental health festival for users, organized by the national association We Shall Overcome (WSO) in collaboration with other mental health organizations. The leader of WSO, Mette Ellingsdalen, had asked me to contribute to Amalie Days, which I was more than happy to do, but I was also a spectator. There were many powerful stories about approaches that haven't worked and the kinds of desired changes. My eyes filled with tears, some of which I shed several times throughout the course of the day. During one of the breaks I found Mette. She was also moved, and we looked at one another and smiled bravely. "You know, Birgit," Mette said to me, "the problem isn't that we cry too much, but that others cry too little."

I have spoken with many people who receive mental health treatment. These are people who have received help elsewhere before coming to see me, others whom I've met through my collaboration with user organizations, some whom I've met at conferences or other meeting places where professionals and users come together. There are many others whom I've read about online, in the media, or in books. They offer a lot of feedback about what does and doesn't work, what they would like more of, and what they would like less of. Based on all these stories, I am certain that the problem within the mental health care services is not about our having insufficient resources or insufficient expert knowledge. It's about how we execute these services and why we do it.

We do too much of what doesn't work. When in different contexts I bring up the stories about what doesn't work, I am told that I mustn't be so negative, but instead focus on the positive, on everything that is good and all those who receive good treatment. However, such a focus will not lead to advances in our field, because we don't improve by looking at what works. It's not just the odd person or two who receive treatment which either doesn't work or even makes things worse. There are many such cases. If we dare enter this space, we won't need more resources. On the contrary: we will presumably manage with fewer.

It might seem difficult to relate to all the obvious kinds of feedback. There is something strange that happens to people when we begin talking about the serious errors that are made within the mental health care sector. I discussed this with Hege Orefellen, a lawyer and a member of WSO. Hege was committed involuntarily in 2003, something she personally feels constituted a violation of her rights, but she wasn't heard, not by the Norwegian Board of Health or by the Parliamentary Ombudsman. She persisted, however, and took legal action. In the end, the health care enterprise was found guilty of several violations of the European Convention on Human Rights. Orefellen's story was told through a documentary which aired on the programme Brennpunkt on the Norwegian television network NRK in the autumn of 2008. The documentary ought to have created waves within the Norwegian mental health care sector. I personally remember being profoundly shaken when I saw it and thought that this would have to have consequences for subsequent practice all over the country. The response was one of complete silence. "What happened afterwards?" I asked. "Did the ruling and the documentary have any consequences?" She smiled and looks at me: "Nothing happened." For her own part, Orefellen found it difficult to understand how the public health service could go on in this way, because she didn't believe the people who work within it want to hurt or violate the rights of patients. Nonetheless, good intentions are not much use when the consequences are so negative for those in question. The mental health care sector continues steadily onward, unperturbed by the feedback. What is it about the mental health care field that neither politicians nor other decision makers who can lead to real changes in the practice dare to have the really tough discussions?

Obvious feedback is often brushed off as being anecdotal. The powers that be insist we need systematic studies, research, something more concrete. The experiences of users don't count here. Instead we look at user surveys or RCT studies, but they don't give us the feedback the field needs. We must start listening, one person at a time, to those who really have something to tell us. We have so much to learn, if we would only dare to take in the negative feedback that's already available out in the open. We must listen; only then will we know what we must do in the way of changes that will work.

Causes of mental health problems – is it really that difficult?

When we really listen, incredible things can happen. We can see what is important to people. Two women, Nina and Beate, have taught me something about this. I had the opportunity to visit the cosy red house where they live together with their four-year-old daughter. They have found peace here. They feel that they have landed and that things are falling into place. It hasn't always been that way. They both have experiences from their childhoods that marked them, and they went many rounds with the public assistance system before I got to know them.

Beate was a real tomboy as a child. She came across as being brave, but Beate told me that inside she felt very small and vulnerable. She was not seen much at home. Her father had been strict and angry a lot, and she doesn't remember much about her mother. She was always told that she wasn't good enough and she could never cry in front of her parents. Beate had a tough exterior, while she always complied with the wishes of her parents. She said she wished somebody had picked up on the fact that she had a desperate need for nurturance and love, although she expressed the opposite. Nina tells me that she never had the chance to be a child; she was the caregiver for her mother and siblings. When the children were upset, they were not allowed to cry, otherwise they would be given a beating. Her mother sometimes took the knife and cut off a birch branch and then they had to line up and receive their punishment one by one. Nina was tough as a child, but over time became quite introverted. She did not seek contact with other children, but played instead by herself. At school, she couldn't concentrate and had little interest in what they were talking about. She had to make sure there was food at home, that the clothing was in order, and that the house was spick and span. She was often underestimated, and many people thought she was dumb. In fact, she was extremely quick-witted from an early age. Nina told me about how she had to think quickly to manage herself in some situations, and several times she saved her mother's life. She wasn't more than seven or eight years old when she walked alone through the city of Trondheim in the middle of the night, searching for her mother so she could bring her home and sober her up.

Nina and Beate understand what was needed for them in order to achieve well-being. "What we yearn for all the time," she said,

> is the nurturance and love we didn't receive when we were young. This isn't available in public health services. There, everything goes according to a script. There are no feelings present, and our feelings are blocked. So we sit there and talk across a table, when maybe it's actually a hug I need the most in order to calm down. I need to be met with comprehension for why I'm is having such a hard time, and not a focus on what's written on a piece of paper. They are extremely hung up on diagnoses. So there are all kinds of things you should and shouldn't do, and then a lot of medication along with it. We're not met as fellow human beings. The therapists need to lighten up on their professional demeanour. In dealing with people, they shouldn't be so unfeeling. I found an alternative therapist who sees me in a completely different way. I have achieved more with her in three months than in six years at DPS [the district psychiatric centre]. It's difficult to explain what she does, but I don't believe they would have managed it at DPS. There are too many forms there, this thick stack of papers about everything that's wrong with me. And I know that when I answer these questions, I will score a little on absolutely all of their diagnoses. And then they offer you a very limited number of sessions. But straightening out 35 years of damage is not done in 10 sessions.

Beate also highlighted compassion, understanding, and equality.

> Throughout our entire lives we have gone around feeling like we are not worth anything, and then we enter a system that makes us feel the same thing. When I was committed, there was an incredible pressure on me to move out of my parents' house and get a job. This was always what they wanted to talk to me about. I knew that I couldn't manage to do that then, so I just felt like even more of a failure. Now, fortunately, I have found a therapist in the local municipal service who has helped me enormously. She has given me the confidence to be myself, wholly and fully. She is there no matter what, and I know that she is fond of me regardless of what I do. She stands by me, accompanying me down this road, and she puts up with me, not because she must but because she wants to. It is a relationship that is more compassionate. At DPS, the first week you're there you're told that you can't use the services here for very long. You feel indebted to them for being there. This is how many sessions you are worth. The therapist in the municipal service sees this differently. She's always there, and just knowing that helps. It has been a lifesaver for me. I have grown from it, and I'm doing much better today.

There are many things that work, and many things that do damage. Nina grew worse from all the tests, the diagnoses, and the focus on what was wrong with her. For Beate, the pressure to find work and her own place to live did not help. The point is that we don't know in advance what will help an individual client. Mental health problems are not definitive entities. There is no scientific basis determining when a mental health disorder arises. Where is the line determining whether or not someone has a disorder, and who will decide this? For some people their current difficulties will clearly be the result of the negligence of adults in their childhood, while for others it may be a combination of many small events combined with their own vulnerability, which make everything complicated. There are many different reasons for why people find themselves struggling. Biological factors also contribute, but when working with healing the context is much more important. I mentioned this in Chapter 6 when in discussing how we to define the market and Bruce Wampold's research on what produces change in therapy. The majority of therapists know this, but nonetheless it appears that research and treatment within a natural science perspective offers greater prestige, and there is more money to be found there. For that reason, a lot of the research is done within this paradigm. Many also believe that identifying biological causes for mental health disorders will make them more acceptable in society, and the stigma will be diminished. But is this actually the case?

More about life and less about illness

When you listen to one person at a time, you discover that their problems are more about life and less about illness. A related issue is how to counteract the stigmatization of people with mental health problems, because influences how we understand them. Sigrun Tømmerås taught me a lot about stigmatization. This subject was not addressed in any way during my education. Since I completed my studies, I have met few professionals who have been particularly interested in the subject, but Tømmerås is. On her blog and Twitter, she posts articles and links to materials that address the subject. A literature search of Tømmerås provided a lot of reading materials and opportunity to learn about mental health and stigmatization.

For Tømmerås, it started in 2004 with an article in the Norwegian newspaper *Dagbladet*, in which she addressed the problem of stigmatization. The article was a response to Greta Ericson and Ann Færden's feature article about incorrect use of psychiatric diagnoses on the part of public individuals and the media as the cause of the problem of stigmatization. Tømmerås highlighted the fact that diagnoses found in nature, but rather contextualized constructions that change in accordance with the time's prevailing customs and conceptions of right and wrong. If Ericson and Færden were concerned about stigmatization, they should instead be interested in how the people who come into contact with psychiatry feel stigmatized by the psychiatrists and psychologists' very diagnoses. Tømmerås (2010) concludes that there is reason to believe that people who are struggling with their lives would be better off if psychiatry brought its diagnostics craze to an end. She is probably right.

Stigmatization takes place when we disqualify people from full social acceptance by assigning them to a classification as deviants. This can lead to individuals being made invisible or marginalized in society and stigmatized groups acquiring a social status that overshadows their other characteristics. The most common way to combat stigma within mental health has been through information and openness about mental health disorders. The thinking has been that prejudices against mental health disorders can be counteracted through increasing understanding. If we could understand the causes behind mental health ailments, we would put an end to prejudices and stigmatization. This is the premise behind most anti-stigma campaigns. The most common approach to informing about and combating stigmatization has been to compare mental health disorders with some type of physical illness.

John Read, now a professor at the University of Liverpool, has spoken out against what he calls the "mental illness is like all other illnesses" approach, an understanding of mental health ailments as biological illnesses "in the brain" (Read, 2007). The thinking behind this approach suggests that, instead of blaming a person for their mental health problems, we might view the symptoms as being a consequence of biological illnesses over which the person has no control. By expanding knowledge about the disorders and more openness, the idea is that it will be easier for people with mental health disorders to seek out treatment. Consequently, there could be a decline in negative stereotypes of people with mental health ailments and greater social acceptance for people with mental health ailments. State institutions, professional organizations, and user organizations support the "mental illness is like all other illness" approach.

Has this approach actually contributed to reducing the stigma? In the article "Evolution of public attitudes about mental illness: a systematic review and meta-analysis", Schomerus and his colleagues (Schomerus, Schwahn, Holzinger, et al., 2012) tried to answer this question. They found that two developments had occurred with respect to the perception of mental illness. One of these was that the population's knowledge about mental illness had increased and that more people sought help. However, the attitudes towards people with mental health disorders had not changed for the better and had even grown worse for people with the diagnosis of schizophrenia. They conclude that a more biological understanding of mental illness has not led to increased social acceptance for people suffering from these illnesses.

Read wanted to understand why biological causal explanations contribute to an increase in prejudices. He referred to Australian research which finds that, when people believe something is based on biology, this represents something uncontrollable. These convictions constitute, according to Read, a dangerous combination. In the article, Read suggested that other research found that we have a greater tendency to assume a condescending attitude towards people with mental health disorders. The less we believe that people are responsible for their actions, the more harshly we treat them, and the less aware we are of our behaviour. Another factor is that we have a need to defend ourselves from madness, and therefore foster an understanding of how people with mental health ailments are a categorically different group of people, instead of all of us sharing a common humanity.

If a biological understanding has a negative impact on how we view people with mental health disorders, how does it affect those who have these problems? Bruce G. Link and his colleagues (Link, Struening, Neese-Todd, Asmussen, & Phelan, 2001) show how stigmatization can impede healing because it impacts self-esteem. Self-esteem is our knowledge and experience of who we are. Self-esteem is about how well we know ourselves and how we relate to what we know. Low self-esteem feels like a constant sense of insecurity, self-critique, and guilt. The researchers found that stigmatization has a strong negative impact on self-esteem. The size of this connection was surprising and cause for concern. Patrick Corrigan (2004) found that people with mental health disorders often internalize the stigmatization and that they personally believe that they are less worthy owing to their mental illness. This, in turn, leads to lower self-esteem and self-efficacy. Evidently, such thoughts can become a barrier to quality of life and goals one might pursue.

There are other ways to understand mental health problems. John Read (2007) says that looking at "psychiatric symptoms" as understandable psychological or emotional reactions to life events, reduces fear, distance, and discrimination. It is also speaking the same language as those who are having difficulties, instead of using professional terminology that is alienating. The most effective way to reduce stigmatization is to know somebody who is experiencing mental health difficulties. By having contact with people with mental health problems outside the treatment situation, the them-and-us divide can be reduced. Many of us have experienced mental health problems to varying degrees. However, when researchers look for biological causes for mental health disorders, they contribute to the distinction between us and them, because even those of us who have experienced mental health problems will think that some mental health ailments are more biological than others, and that these are categorically different. I have spoken with many people who allegedly have the most serious mental health problems. Even though these can manifest as being extremely biological in nature, many of these people are convinced that the combination of life events with their own vulnerability caused them to react as they have done.

The book *Drøm i våken tilstand* ("Dreaming While Awake") (Kristiansen, Rydheim, & Thyness, 2013) offers a good example of how one acquires a broader understanding of mental health problems by reading the accounts of those who have experienced them. The book includes seven stories told by people who have experienced psychosis. In the epilogue, author Merete Morken Andersen writes (p. 179):

> One listens to a lived story in a different way than when one reads an evidence-based research article. ... when the listening muscle starts to become agile and well-tuned, a new form of energy enters the experience, one that opens us up to moving forward, passing through that which has grown rigid, and the world can expand with greater nuance.

We probably need more such stories to loosen up the medical stock language and dare to trust that one can help more through genuine contact and proximity than through procedures, scientific distance, and control.

What can we learn from the feedback from users?

Our field provides us with feedback all the time. We can acquire this through systematic registration procedures, such as the use of FIT or other methods, and if we open ourselves to receive it. We must take in all these stories and learn from them. We should thank all the patients, clients, and users who try to tell us something, even though it may be about something we need to change. We must remember that while it can be difficult to receive negative feedback, it is even more difficult to give it, particularly if the user is unsure about whether the feedback will be welcomed.

Many signs suggest that an understanding of psychological problems based on diagnoses and biological illness is not adequate. Perceiving psychological problems as an illness doesn't leads to reduced stigmatization but, rather, the opposite. Why then do we continue developing services based on such a conceptual framework? Shouldn't we have learned something by now?

Methods are heaped upon us that supposedly will tell us how we can better help people who are having difficulties. One method surpasses the next, and there are constantly new tools and protocols to adopt and learn. There is an idea in the field that, if the professionals would only apply the right methods to the correctly diagnosed problems, we will witness advancement and development. That is not always true. We need to approach the development of the field in another way. We must be less concerned about what we should do and more focused on understanding the process of how we arrive at the correct procedure. Mental health care services of the future require a new way of thinking, one that will advance the field.

We can't solve our problems by using the same thinking we used when we created them.

Albert Einstein

8

BEYOND BEST PRACTICE

We must not cease from exploration, and the end of all our exploring will be to arrive where we began and to know the place for the first time.

T.S. Eliot

In March 2013, Stangehelp in Stange received a wonderful visit. When State Secretary Kjell Erik Øie from the Norwegian Ministry of Health and Care Services went to the president of the Norwegian Psychologists Association, Tor Levin Hofgaard, and wanted advice on where he should ask about good outcomes in the field of mental health care, the answer was clear: Go to Stange! Hofgaard was familiar with how we work at Stangehelp. Together with the state secretary he came from Oslo to hear a presentation. The day arrived, we were all dressed up, and the table in the meeting room was decorated with flowers. I started by telling him about our service, the principles according to which we work, and the results we achieved. Øie was visibly impressed. At one point, he asked me, "But what is it you actually do?" I looked at him and hesitated. I didn't know how to answer that question. A bit flustered, I managed to say, "We do many different things," and gave a few vague examples.

After the guests left, I continued to think about this question. It bothered me that I hadn't given a better response. Why hadn't I prepared myself better? That was a natural question. I considered these thoughts as I drove back and forth to work, and one day it came to me. The reason I wasn't able to answer the question was because it was the wrong question. The question State Secretary Øie should have asked was: how do you work out what you should do?

It isn't important to explain what we do, but rather the process that leads us to what we do. If we understand this process, we will also understand how to work on the basis of the feedback we receive and our reflections about it. It is the learning process that is important. We learn the multiplication tables by heart, but if we don't understand the concept of multiplication we haven't actually learned anything about arithmetic. We have just memorized some numbers. That is also how it is in our field. We can always learn a few methods, but if we don't understand the process of determining what we need to do, when, and with whom then we haven't learned anything about change work. We can only learn about this one family at a time, one service at a time, and one municipality at a time.

Accumulated knowledge

I presented these ideas at a conference in Amsterdam in May 2013. Scott Miller and his colleagues arranged the Achieving Clinical Excellence conference for the second time, and I was to give a presentation about how we work according to a deliberate practice mentality at Stangehelp in Stange. Accordingly: how do we arrive at what we are going to do? This book, thus far, has already offered the answer, but one of the guests at the conference challenged me. K. Anders Ericsson was the keynote speaker, but he also listened to all of our presentations. During the breaks, I had the opportunity to enjoy a number of good conversations with Ericsson, and I heard his views on our way of implementing deliberate practice. This was his concept and his area of expertise.

Ericsson has little experience with the field of psychotherapy, but he asked me whether I had any accumulated knowledge to offer from our work. Other fields, such as chess, mathematics, and music, have advanced because there is some knowledge about which everyone agrees. For example, when one is going to learn to play the piano, all the keys have a name and there is some fundamental knowledge about how to read music and move one's fingers across the keys. Ericsson challenged me to think through whether this kind of accumulated knowledge exists within the field of mental health care and, if so, what it would consist of. He shared my concerns that, if therapists only learn methods they can employ in specific situations, they won't be prepared to generate and use more general procedures that may be fundamental to becoming proficient in the long term.

Does such accumulated knowledge exist within the field of mental health care? I find that sometimes we are virtually unable to agree about anything within this field. We can't even agree about what mental health problems are. I called Scott Miller again, to discuss this with him. Miller said there are two things we can agree upon: the client's engagement and the negotiation over the alliance. Orlinsky, Rønnestad, and Willutzki (2004) highlight the client's engagement in the change process as being the most important factor for achieving change. There is a broad consensus in the profession about the alliance being a factor of critical important to improvement and that this must form the basis for the work. Engagement and alliance are where we must begin; there are few who will argue against this. How one does this is up to the individual, but the goal must be to engage the client in his own improvement process, and that is best achieved by forming a good work alliance.

Miller also discussed the problems with the way in which we develop our competence:

> Within psychotherapy we have reached a point where we teach therapists very many different models. Eventually, one discovers that the method one has learned is not adequate, and one begins on a long and convoluted journey to develop one's skills. Many then end up with the *messy house syndrome*. One has actually not set any goals when one

> decorates one's house, one just collects a lot of things (or methods) which one puts all over the house. When somebody comes to visit they say "Oh, how interesting, Oh how interesting, Oh how interesting." But if anyone should ask about the overriding theme of the house, there is just a lot of clutter there, and no common theme. And if you ask a person with a messy house for one specific thing, the person will not be able to find it. And often he has maybe five of the same thing, but he can't find them and neither does he know how they are used. Many therapists end up here. They collect methods over time, and they don't even know what they know. This stands in contrast to those who end up with a house that has a theme. They start with the fundamental things one needs in a house. And since they reflect upon how they want the house to be, they don't end up with a house full of clutter. If things don't serve their intended purpose, you don't hang onto them. You might find them interesting, but you don't save them. And if they do serve their intended purpose, then one asks under which conditions they do so. This beautiful object belongs in the kitchen and not in the bathroom.

I told Miller about my two eldest children, who had just started taking piano lessons. My son, who learns things by heart very quickly, could probably have learned a quite difficult piece by memorizing the notes and without needing to have the basic skills first. However, by doing it in this way, he wouldn't actually know how to play the piano. My daughter, who likes to experiment and learns through trial and error, would never have gone along with such a process. She wants to develop knowledge through a natural learning process and doesn't take shortcuts to become good at something.

Miller understood the comparison right away. "The same is true for therapy," he said:

> or to use another term, change work. We can all learn methods and models, but that doesn't mean we master the art of doing change work. Some of the best pianists can play pieces within their genre extremely well, and when they are exposed to a special context, they can vary a bit; they know exactly the type of knowledge or skill they must use there and then.

So what can we agree upon within therapy? The client's engaged participation is the objective. Therapists who have this objective in mind will eventually learn to structure the work better in order to accomplish this. The therapist learns what serves this purpose and reflects upon what he or she does. Thus, they won't end up with a lot of methods which when combined just create a mess with no overview. This is not about learning a theoretical approach, but about how to handle and organize the work of negotiating an alliance between therapist and client, as well as the structure surrounding this process.

Back to the beginning – simplicity and complexity

Consider the story about LEGO in Chapter 6. LEGO virtually doubled the number of its components in seven years. The designers' free rein resulted in the creation of increasingly complex models, wholly out of sync with what children wanted. The designers thought it was exciting and were allowed to do as they pleased. The staff weren't concerned about the company's success, but about producing models that they found exciting. This almost led to the company's downfall.

The number of methods within the field of mental health care has exploded in the past 50 years without this leading to real advancement. Advancement requires novel approaches and innovation. True innovation changes the course of the field and leads to value creation in the long run. Unfortunately, innovation is often confused with variation. Simon Sinek uses Colgate as an example of this in his book *Start with Why*. In the 1970s, there were just two types of Colgate toothpaste. Eventually, as the competition increased, sales began to decline. The company then introduced a new product, with a new feature, and another one, then another one, and then another one. Each new product helped the sales figures at least for a little while. Today you can choose between 32 different types of Colgate toothpaste. Since the other companies respond to Colgate's "innovation" in kind, they offer the same number of varieties with approximately the same quality at approximately the same price. There are dozens of different types of toothpastes to choose from, but there is no data demonstrating that we brush our teeth more now than we did in the 1970s. Thanks to all this innovation it is now virtually impossible to determine which type of toothpaste is right for you.

Coming up with yet another therapy method that is similar to what we already have, but with a new twist here and there, is not innovation. Inventing new methods is fine, but usually this doesn't represent innovation, only variation. Something new does not necessarily add to the field. It's only a new way of doing more of the same.

If the field is to move forward, we must expand our knowledge in another way. Our interest must be in what works, starting with a practice-based approach. Let me tell a story about a man who was concerned about results. Hungarian physician Ignatz Semmelweis was the man who pioneered the notion that doctors should wash their hands. The mortality rate of maternity patients was extremely high at the end of the 19th century, and Semmelweis's theory was that, if doctors washed their hands with bleach, the mortality rate would go down. He did a study that achieved fantastic results. The mortality rate dropped by all of 90%. He published his results, but the rest of the medical community did not want to listen to him because they wanted to know *why*. Semmelweis couldn't provide an acceptable scientific explanation for why handwashing helped. It wasn't evidence-based. Semmelweis didn't care about that; he just wanted to prevent women from dying in childbirth. He was interested in outcomes.

Change work is sometimes about doing things in the simplest way, and understanding that the simple way is often the best way. In order to truly excel, however, we must also understand complexity. We need to understand all the nuances of the challenges people are facing in order to know exactly the type of knowledge to use in a given circumstance.

Think for yourself

It is the employees who make the service outstanding. We must enable individuals to perform at their very best in order to provide overall good service. This means individual employees must develop in ways that they can make independent decisions within specified guidelines, fundamental principles, and the feedback that comes in along the way. In their book *Practical Wisdom – The Right Way to Do the Right Thing*, Barry Schwartz and Kenneth Sharpe (2010) have explored this in detail. They draw connections all the way back to Aristotle's teachings about practical wisdom, which include the moral will to do what is right and the moral skills to find out what this is. What this means is that we must find the right way to do what is right in a specific situation with a specific person at a given moment. Aristotle claimed that achieving this requires practical wisdom.

For most of what we work with in mental health care, there is no single solution for everyone. Rules and procedures can help us to a certain extent and serve as guidelines, but they will never be nuanced enough to help us in every situation. Aristotle maintained that finding a balance for this required wisdom, and this had to be practical because the questions we usually meet are found in our daily work. Being wise means, according to Aristotle, that we have the right purpose or intentions for the work we are going to do, which he called *telos*. Every occupational group has a *telos*, whether in banking or social work, and a good practitioner is manages to find his or her *telos* and work towards it. It requires practical wisdom to be able to translate the objective into action. It is not enough simply to have good intentions. That's where we got the adage: the road to hell is paved with good intentions. The answer to the question "What shall I do?" almost always depends upon the specifics of the situation.

Schwartz and Sharpe challenge our assumptions when we attempt to make improvements, specifically in the area of rules and incentives. Rules and administrative control mechanisms tell people what to do and how to monitor their performance in order to ensure that their actions are in compliance with the regulations. Incentives also encourage performance excellence by offering rewards. There is no doubt that we need some rules and incentives in our services. We need rules to protect us from disaster and people have to earn a living. At the same time, however, rules without wisdom are blind and can at best guarantee mediocrity. As Daniel Pink taught us in Chapter 6, too many incentives will actually deprive us of the motivation to excel.

Schwartz and Sharpe claim that a wise person knows when he can break the rules and when he must improvise. Wise people evolve; they are not born that way. We have every opportunity to become wise, but then we need experience that allows us to proceed by trial and error. We need continuous feedback on what we do and supervision from wise mentors. Wisdom does not necessarily require grand-scale performances, but without wisdom grand performances will never be enough.

Let's return to the visit of State Secretary Øie. Following Hofgaard's recommendation, he was clear about how the government wanted to invest in mental health care services in the municipalities, but they were struggling to determine how this could be funded in a way that ensured that the best possible quality. "You want to spend money on mental health care in Norway, but at the same time you need to know whether what you are investing money in will actually generate any dividends." I asked Øie, "How are you going to ensure that?" This is a question politicians struggle with, and Øie was unable to come up with a good answer. A lot of money has been allocated to mental health care in recent years, but it is doubtful whether the results have been on a par with the investment. What we need to do is create structures in the organizations that make it possible to work in a way that enables us to develop wisdom rather than suppress it. Rules and incentives are demoralizing, which is something psychological research has known for 30 years.

When we suppress employees' opportunities to make their own assessments and think for themselves, Schwartz and Sharpe (2010) claim that this results in naughty rule-breakers. These are people who manage to find ways of bypassing the rules; they adapt only to the exact degree required to simultaneously maintain the latitude to do what they believe in. The problem is that they can't carry on like this for long and will eventually give up. On the other hand, there are the system changers. These don't try to subvert the rules but instead try to change the system. They succeed in doing so in some cases, particularly in small-scale contexts and where there is a lot of local decision-making authority. In the final analysis, people want to be allowed to do what is right, because that also makes them happier.

What will progress look like?

If someone had succeeded in creating structures within organizations to secure the type of processes described by Schwartz and Sharpe (2010) and as I have described in this book, how then would our field have developed? What would we have filled it with? What kind of results would we achieve?

I was fortunate enough to hear Ingebrigt Steen Jensen speak about Rosenborg, the soccer team from Trondheim, which is illustrated in detail in his book *Ona fyr* (Jensen, 2002). The stories goes as follows: Nils Arne Eggen, a high school teacher from Orkdal, took over the team with one goal in sight. Rosenborg was to become Europe's best soccer club team. His starting point was a small team in a small city where it snows for six months out of the year and the rain falls horizontally for the other six. Eggen wanted to use mainly local boys from the towns of Melhus, Ranheim, and Kyrkjsæterøra. With this as his point of departure, he would in less than 10 years create one of the best soccer teams in Europe. Such a plan sounds ludicrous, but Eggen managed it, because under Eggen's leadership Rosenborg was a visionary and value-driven team that understood what leads to success.

Eggen has been generous about explaining what he did at Rosenborg. He wrote a book, held lectures, and spoke with other coaches about their methods. Jensen, a Stabæk enthusiast, once had a conversation with Eggen about this. "When you are so open about what you do, aren't you afraid that others will do the same, so that we become just as good or even better than your team?" Eggen replied, "That doesn't concern me, because by the time you start doing what we are doing, we will have begun doing something else."

Eggen knew how to arrive at the answer for what one should do, which is more important than copying what others do. For that reason, Jensen also says that it was impossible to copy Rosenborg. If somebody contacts me and wants to learn about how we work in Stange, I am not particularly concerned with telling them about what we do. I don't list methods, measures, or other things we have used along the way, because if they simply start copying this they will have missed the entire point. It's not what we do that is important; it's how we find out what we should do that I try to communicate to visitors. By the time they've started doing what we do, it could be that we have started doing something else. Perhaps we have replaced the couch, because it is no longer suitable in the living room or other needs have arisen. Perhaps we have rearranged or acquired new furniture. Our house is also tailored for Stange municipality. It might be out of place in Bærum or Hammerfest. They might need a different type of architecture and other kinds of furniture. Everyone must find out for themselves how to furnish their own homes. However, it is generally safe to assume that everyone needs the most fundamental things, such as a floor, a roof, and walls. Everybody wants a kitchen and bathroom.

We must accept that we can't know now how our field will appear in the future. If we make huge plans, create projects, and believe in advance that we know what the outcome will be, we will probably miss out on the great discoveries that will occur along the way. Basically, we cannot predict what the future will bring. In his book *Ripples from the Zambezi* (1999), Sirolli says (although he isn't sure whether it is true) that in 1860 a group of psychics were asked to predict what the city of New York would look like in 100 years. Everyone agreed that by 1960 the city of New York would no longer exist, owing to population growth. The population would be so large that six million horses would be required to transport all the people around the city. They surmised that horse dung from six million horses would have created such a large problem that the residents would be forced to leave the city.

We cannot predict the future. We do our best to develop strategies and plans in an effort to predict the outcomes. Our challenge becomes growing through the complexity of the work we do and accepting the uncertainty required to discover something we could not see in advance. By developing the field based on doing something that works, we may eventually anticipate something other than horse dung.

Paradigms

If you want to make minor, incremental changes and improvements, work on practices, behavior, or attitude. But if you want to make significant, quantum improvement, work on paradigms.

Stephen R. Covey

In *The Seven Habits of Highly Effective People* (1989), Stephen R. Covey explains how our paradigms affect our behaviour, which in turn affects our results. The word paradigm is actually a scientific term meaning a model, theory, notion, assumption, or frame of reference. In general, it is how we see the world, based on our understanding and interpretations. One analogy might be to think of paradigms as maps, and we all know that maps are not the terrain. A map is a clarification of specific aspects of the terrain, and that is also how it is for paradigms. They are a theory, an explanation of something else.

Since the term paradigm is related to science, we might not always think about its influence on our daily lives. However, the way we look at, understand and interpret the world – our mental map – will inevitably influence what we do. We all walk around with internal paradigms that control the way we act. Our actions result in our accomplishing something; we achieve a result from what we do. If the results do not fully live up to what we had in mind, we return to our behaviour, trying to adjust it in hopes of bringing about improvements. For a while we may succeed, but in seeking only to change external actions and attitudes we accomplish little in the long run, as long as we fail to investigate the fundamental paradigms from which these actions stem.

Paradigm shifts is a concept that was introduced by Thomas Kuhn in *The Structure of Scientific Revolutions* (1962). He suggested that all important scientific breakthroughs are first a break with tradition, old mentalities, and established paradigms. We can also experience small paradigm shifts in our daily lives – moments when we see things differently – and this influences our entire manner of relating to something. The more attached we are to our own notions and conceptions (paradigms), the more dramatic the moment of epiphany will be when we begin to see things differently. It's like turning on a light bulb. Consider the research of Daryl Chow presented in Chapter 5. It was the therapists who were the most surprised by feedback who not only changed the most, but who achieved the best outcomes. However, as human beings it can be hard for us to change our understandings and interpretations because it means letting go of something we thought was real or true.

If we succeed in evaluating our paradigms and moving from one view of the world to another, it can produce sweeping changes, whether the shift occurs in the wink of an eye or through a slow, well-considered process.

What do we want for the field of mental health care?

I have already written about this in Chapter 4, and I will repeat it now: Mental health issues are a large problem in society. For example, in Norway, they 60–70 billion kroner per year. While illness absenteeism is otherwise on the decline, the number of people on sick leave owing to mental health ailments is on the rise. Researchers report that mental health disorders are a main cause of illness absenteeism and disability – and this particularly true for young people. Half the young people who receive disability benefits do so owing to mental health ailments. Everyone agrees that steps must be taken to do something about these problems.

In Norway, as in many other locations, the response has been money and services. The belief is that channelling more money into public services or establishing new services will solve the problems. However, the new services create new problems, so more efforts must be established to address the new problems. This leads to reorganization, sometimes on a large scale, such as the reforms of the Norwegian Labor and Welfare Organization (NAV) and the Coordination Reform, while other reform measures have been on a smaller scale. Unfortunately, innovative thinking can be rare. There is no basis in new underlying values and no vision to strive for. It's a matter of economics and service production in different packaging. The problems in locations such as Norway will not be solved by more money or more public services. If that were the case, we would not have any problems in Norway.

What we need is a new and different way of thinking about mental health care services. Stephen R. Covey (1989) says, "We see the world, not as it is, but as *we* are – or, as we are conditioned to see it. … The way we see the problems *is* the problem."

We need structures in organizations that will make it possible to think in new and different ways in order to develop approaches based on feedback from clients. Then we must be willing and disciplined enough to let go of those things that aren't effective and may even be detrimental. That requires courage on the part of health care politicians and health care leaders, but it is possible.

The mental health services of the future

The place to improve the world is first in one's own heart and head and hands, and then work outward from there.

Robert Pirsig

On a warm summer day in 2013, I was sitting on a bench beneath the sweltering sun and looking out across the grounds of the Hagen treatment centre. Andy, my first mentor, sat beside me, and we talked about the time that had passed since I sat here for the first time eight years earlier. The grass lawn where children can run around was the same, as was the traditional Norwegian storehouse, the swings, and the apple orchard below. Andy was among the first in Norway to implement systematic feedback from clients, long before others had begun thinking along those lines. I asked him what prompted him to start doing this.

> It was around the time when R.E.M. came out with the song "Losing My Religion". I was struggling with what we were doing at Hagen and asked myself all the time whether we were actually doing anything that was truly helpful. I was working with a boy, whom I had assumed responsibility for "saving", but I was absolutely not saving him, even though I had a good understanding of and belief in the prevailing treatment theory and practice of the time. I was in the process of destroying myself and the boy was not experiencing any improvement. We kept young people in treatment for such a long time and it was difficult to know when we were finished. There were so many things I had doubts about. We invested so much and even though I believe that many were doing well, I was on the verge of losing faith in the work we were doing. I wanted to improve, to achieve better outcomes from our work. I wanted what we were doing to work! That people would succeed in changing their lives, that they would feel better. It was that simple.

Andy was seeking new knowledge. At a conference in 1994, he came across *Changing the Rules* by Duncan, Solovey, and Rusk (1992). The book appealed to Andy very much. It offered something he had been searching for to improve his practice and enable him to help people properly. When he returned to Hagen, he asked for permission to do things differently. At first, he was allowed to carry out a different type of admission process with one family. Previous admission procedures were extremely formal processes in which they read all the papers and subsequently all the professionals sat down to decide what was going to be done. Andy was now allowed to convene the involved parties, including the mother, and arrange a meeting, during which he interviewed all of them.

> Everyone sat around a big table, psychologist, social worker, child welfare representatives, and people from the school system. The mother sat directly facing me with her head virtually down between her knees and I thought: "Good Lord, what have I done!" It was terrifying, and I didn't exactly have the support of the professionals surrounding me. Many of them were sceptical, but I was allowed to proceed. I asked the mother: "Why did you agree to allow them to refer your son to us?" Then she looked up at me and said that in fact she did not agree. Then I asked her what it was that she could believe in, what she thought would help the most. She lifted her head, and eventually she dominated the entire meeting. We decided on a treatment plan there and then. Little by little, the mother began sitting up straight. That was how it started.

For Andy this was revolutionary. This reversal of power in the change process and its administration has been a provocation for many professionals and it has incited many reactions. "But I had to find something that could show results. And then I found it. Or it found me. That book called to me!" I asked Andy why he thought some people became very interested in this, while others dismissed it.

> It's hard to say. This wasn't just something I did on a hunch. It was founded on solid research and well substantiated, but it is very challenging for our systems. It told the system that they must do something differently. A lot of the resistance can be about fear: the fear of doing something wrong, of failure, or fear of the culture in which one is working. If you go against a system, it strikes back. Unlike individuals, the system has no conscience or own objective. Systems perpetuate themselves. If you threaten a system, something happens. I was told that I had over-identified with my clients and that I should get counselling to address this. At Hagen, we would eventually not have meetings without including the clients, but many professionals wanted the professionals to come to an agreement first among themselves before meeting the clients. But why should five or six professionals reach a consensus and subsequently appear as a power front when they meet with this one person who was suffering? And why did we have to agree? Can't people benefit from our differences of opinion, so they have a choice?

Andy has been doing this for a long time. He has seen methods come and go. "I'm completely sure that it isn't about the method. I became very adept at some methods, but I saw that they didn't work for everyone." I asked what he would change within the field of mental health care, based on all the feedback he has received over the years.

> First and foremost, I would abandon the medical model as the primary provider for the structure of mental health care, with respect to direct therapeutic work, administration, and research. In our field, the medical paradigm has no scientific basis. It is fundamentally based on tradition rather than knowledge. At the same time, this paradigm is fixed by law. Ideally, we should do away with the law so that a specified group of professionals are no longer given priority when it comes to defining how we should go about helping people, without including people's own expertise and engagement. That means a different type of assistance scheme which supports the clients' own processes.

Andy doesn't actually believe that the art of helping people is so complicated.

> We know a lot about the art of helping and we must believe in people's ability to help themselves and each other. We have to believe in people's own competence. Helping each other is a human quality, it is not something academic or something one group of professionals does better than another. This is something people have done throughout the ages, but when we turn the work of helping people into a profession, expectations arise, both in ourselves and others about what we have "created". These expectations will potentially exercise power over us and result in our being controlled or tied to our "creation". We identify with what we have done, and a wish arises to preserve what we have been working with for so long. That simultaneously leads to uneasiness because we have no control over the perspectives of others and accordingly their ideas about and expectations of us. Strong discipline is required in order to let go of something one has been working on for a long time, because our self-esteem and personal well-being is invested in what we have "created".

"In the end isn't it about helping people so they can start doing something themselves that is good for them?" I asked.

> Yes. Each meeting with a human being is new. What those of us who are helpers need is to learn what motivates and gives our clients opportunities to move forward in their lives. This applies to us as therapists, but also to how we organize our services.

Then we must have the courage to let go of something, in order to achieve progress.

Then Andy told me the story about the Zen Buddhist.

> Once upon a time, long ago there was a Zen Buddhist monk who was uniquely gifted in painting landscapes. Any exhibition would have been thrilled to include his paintings, but he wanted something different. Instead, he spent time on board a boat that slowly drifted down a winding river. He didn't use oars but allowed the calmly flowing river to guide the boat forward. While he was sitting there, he painted fabulous landscape pictures of the surroundings that revealed themselves around him. When he finished with a painting, he let it slip down into the river, without signing it. Then he started working on a new painting. He did this over and over again as he travelled down the river.

Every day we learn something new, discover something we didn't know before, and challenge established truths. When we really take the time to listen to what people tell us about what they want and what it is that helps them, we begin to see infinitely many possibilities. From here, we start to see just how far this field can go. The potential for helping people in better and more effective ways is quite simply enormous.

A man walking is never in balance but always correcting for imbalance.
Gregory Bateson

EPILOGUE BY BIRGIT VALLA

There was a cork bulletin board hanging in my mother's office in the basement of our home. On this bulletin board hung a card bearing a text titled "The Law of Anti-Jante", and I remember it well. When we read such things while growing up, we start to believe in them. Now it hangs at Stangehelp, both for those who work there and those who drop by.

The law of Anti-Jante

You are unique.
You worth is beyond estimation.
You know how to do something that only you can do.
You have something to give others.
You have done something that you can be proud of.
You have enormous untapped resources.
You are a "good for something."
You can accept others.

You have the ability to understand and learn from others.
There is somebody who loves you.

By Erling Førland

EPILOGUE BY DAVID S. PRESCOTT

Hopefully, the next step after reading this book will be for each reader to establish their own map for professional development, including establishing a baseline of effectiveness and routine monitoring of outcomes and the alliance. Next, this map can involve embarking on a plan of deliberate practice, aided by an expert coach. My personal suggestion is not only to join relevant professional organizations in your specialty areas of practice, but also to become part of the community of FIT practitioners, those who seek to move beyond the currently accepted best practices. There is much to learn from their stories as well.

Good luck on your journey!

REFERENCES

Adolph, K.E., Shrout, P.E., & Vereijken, B. (2003). What changes in infant walking and why. *Child Development*, 74, 475–497.

American Psychiatric Association (1980). *Diagnostic and Statistical Manual of Mental Disorders* (3rd ed.). Washington, DC: American Psychiatric Association.

American Psychiatric Association (2013). *Diagnostic and Statistical Manual of Mental Disorders* (5th ed.). Washington, DC: American Psychiatric Association.

Andersen, A.J.W., & Larsen, I.B. (2012). Hell on earth: Textual reflections on the experience of mental illness. *Journal of Mental Health*, 21, 174–181.

Anker, M., Duncan, B.L., & Sparks, J.A. (2009). Using client feedback to improve couple therapy outcomes: A randomized clinical trial in a naturalistic setting. *Journal of Consulting and Clinical Psychology*, 77, 693–704.

Anker, M.G., Sparks, J.A., Duncan, B.L., Owen, J.J., & Stapnes, A.K. (2011). Footprints of couple therapy: Client reflections at follow-up. *Journal of Family Psychotherapy*, 22(1), 22–45.

Babins-Wagner, R. (2017). FIT in Agency and Clinic Settings. In D.S. Prescott, C.M. Maeschalck, & S.D. Miller (Eds.), *Feedback-Informed Treatment in*

Clinical Practice: Reaching for Excellence (pp. 167–185). Washington, DC: American Psychological Association.

Bergin, A.E. (1978). The Evaluation of Therapeutic Outcomes. In A.E. Bergin & S.L. Garfield (Eds.), *Handbook of Psychotherapy and Behaviour Change* (pp. 941–963). New York: Wiley.

Carroll, L. (1865). *Alice's Adventures in Wonderland*. Norsk Utgave: *Alice I Eventyrland*. Oslo: Aschehoug.

Chow, D. (2014). *The study of supershrinks: Development and deliberate practices of highly effective psychotherapists*. PhD thesis, Curtin University, Australia.

Chow, D.L., Miller, S.D., Seidel, J.A., Kane, R.T., & Thornton, J.A. (2015). The role of deliberate practice in the development of highly effective psychotherapists. *Psychotherapy*, 52, 337–345.

Colvin, G. (2008). *Talent Is Overrated. What Really Separates World-Class Performers from Everybody Else*. London: Nicholas Brealey Publishing.

Corrigan, P. (2004). How stigma interferes with mental health care. *American Psychologist*, 59, 614–625.

Covey, S.R. (1989). *The Seven Habits of Highly Effective People*. London: Simon & Schuster.

Coyle, D. (2009). *The Talent Code. Greatness Isn't Born, It's Grown*. London: Arrow Books.

de Jong, K., van Sluis, P., Nugter, M.A., Heiser, W.J., & Spinhoven, P. (2012). Understanding the differential impact of outcome monitoring: Therapist variables that moderate feedback effects in a randomized clinical trial. *Psychotherapy Research*, 22, 464–474.

Duncan, B.L. (2010). *On Becoming a Better Therapist*. Washington, DC: American Psychological Association.

Duncan, B.L., Miller, S.D., & Sparks, J.A. (2004). *The Heroic Client: A Revolutionary Way to Improve Effectiveness through Client-Directed, Outcome-Informed Therapy*, San Francisco, CA: Jossey-Bass.

Duncan, B.L., Solovey, A.D., & Rusk, G.S. (1992). *Changing the Rules: A Client-Directed Approach to Therapy*. New York: Guilford Press.

Dweck, C.S. (2006). *Mindset. The New Psychology of Success*. New York: Ballantine Books.

Dyregrov, A. (2007). *Sorg hos barn*. Oslo: Fagbokforlaget.

Ekecrantz, L.S. (1995). *Patienternas psykiatri: en studie av institutionella erfarenheter*. Stockholm: Carlsson Bokförlag.

Ekeland, T.J. (2012). Sjelens Ingeniørkunst. Om Psykologien og Psykologenes Selvforståelse. *Tidsskri for Norsk Psykologforening*, 49, 746–752.

Ericsson, K.A. (2006). The Influence of Experience and Deliberate Practice on the Development of Superior Expert Performance. S. 684. In K.A. Ericsson, N. Charness, P.J. Feltovich, & R.R. Hoffman (Eds.), *The Cambridge Handbook of Expertise and Expert Performance* (pp. 698–703). New York: Cambridge University Press.

Ericsson, K.A., Charness, N., Feltovich, P.J., & Hoffman, R.R. (2006). *The Cambridge Handbook of Expertise and Expert Performance*. New York: Cambridge University Press.

Ericsson, K.A., Krampe, R.T., & Tesch-Romer, C. (1993). The role of deliberate practice in the acquisition of expert performance. *Psychological Review*, 100, 363–406.

Ericsson, K.A., & Lehman, A.C. (1996). Expert and exceptional performance: Evidence of maximal adaptation to task constraints. *Annual Review of Psychology*, 47, 273–305.

Eysenck, H.J. (1957). The effects of psychotherapy: An evaluation. *Journal of Consulting Psychology*, 16(5): 319–324.

Eysenck, H.J. (1966). *The Effects of Psychotherapy*. New York: International Science Press.

Friedman, M. (2009). *Trying Hard Is Not Good Enough. How to Produce Measurable Improvements for Customers and Communities*. Charleston, SC: BookSurge Publishing.

Gladwell, M. (2008). *Outliers. The Story of Success*. London: Penguin Books.

Gleave, R.L., Burlingame, G.M., Beecher, M.E., Griner, D., Hansen, K., & Jenkins, S.A. (2017). Feedback-Informed Group Treatment: Application of the OQ-45 and Group Questionnaire. In D.S. Prescott, C.M. Maeschalck, & S.D. Miller (Eds.), *Feedback-Informed Treatment in Clinical Practice: Reaching for Excellence* (pp. 141–166). Washington, DC: American Psychological Association.

Goldacre, B. (2008). *Bad Science: Quacks, Hacks and Big Pharma Flacks*. New York: Faber and Faber, Inc.

Goldberg, S.B., Rousmaniere, T., Miller, S.D., Whipple, J., Nielsen, S.L., Hoyt, W.T., & Wampold, B.E. (2016). Do psychotherapists improve with time and experience? A longitudinal analysis of real world outcome data. *Journal of Consulting and Clinical Psychology*, 63, 1–11.

Hannan, C., Lambert, M.L., Harmon, C., Nielsen, S.L., Smart, D.W., Shimokawa, K., & Sutton, S.W. (2005). A lab test and algorithms for identifying clients at risk for treatment failure. *Journal of Clinical Psychology*, 61, 155–163.

Holte, A. (2012). Forebygg psykiske lidelser. *Dagsavisen*, 8 March 2012. Retrieved from www.dagsavisen.no/nyemeninger/forebygg-psykiske-lidelser-1.441059.

Jensen, I.S. (2002). *Ona fyr (One Lighthouse). For deg som vil lykkes sammen med andre*. Oslo: Dinamo Forlag.

Johnstone, L. (2015). *Straight Talking Introduction to Psychiatric Diagnosis*. Ross-on-Wye, UK: PCCS Books.

Kahneman, D. (2011). *Thinking Fast and Slow*. London: Allen Lane.

Kristiansen, G.H., Rydheim, S.H., & Thyness, E.M. (2013). *Drøm i våken tilstand*. Oslo: Abstrakt forlag.

Kuhn, T. (1962). *The Structure of Scientific Revolutions* Chicago, IL: University of Chicago Press.

Lambert, M.J. (2010). Yes, It Is Time for Clinicians to Routinely Monitor Treatment Outcome. In B. Duncan, S.D. Miller, B.E. Wampold, & M. Hubble (Eds.), *The Heart and Soul of Change. Delivering What Works* (2nd ed.) (pp. 239–266). Washington, DC: American Psychological Association.

Lambert, M.J., Bergin, A.E., & Collins, J.L. (1977). Therapist-Induced Deterioration in Psychotherapy. In A.S. Gurman, & A.M. Razin (Eds.), *Effective Psychotherapy. A Handbook of Research* (pp. 452–481). Exeter: A. Wheaton & Co. Ltd.

Lambert, M.J., Morton, J.J., Hatfield, D., Harmon, C., Hamilton, S., Reid, R.C., et al. (2004). *Administration and Scoring Manual for the Outcome Questionnaire – 45*. Salt Lake City, UT: OQ Measures.

Larsen, I.B., & Andersen, A.J.W. (2011a). En hellig plikt. Hvordan beskriver brukere av psykisk helsevern seg selv, og hvilke motiver oppgir de for å nedfelle sine erfaringer skriflig? *Klinisk sygepleje*, 25, 38–47.

Larsen, I.B., & Andersen, A.J.W. (2011b). Tvangstrøye og ensomhet, blomstervaser og kjærlighet. Hvordan beskriver skandinaviske brukere av psykisk helsevern sine erfaringer med den hjelpen de ble tilbudt? *Tidsskrift for psykisk helsearbeid*, 8, 120–130.

Lemow, D., Woolway, E., & Yezzi, K. (2012). *Practice Perfect. 42 Rules for Getting Better at Getting Better*. San Francisco, CA: Jossey-Bass.

Levitt, T. (1960). *Marketing Myopia*. Retrieved from https://hbr.org/2004/07/marketing-myopia.

Link, B.G., Struening, E.L., Neese-Todd, S., Asmussen, S., & Phelan, J.C. (2001). The consequences of stigma for the self-esteem of people with mental illnesses. *Psychiatric Services*, 52, 1621–1626.

Luborsky, L. (1954). A note on Eysenck's article "The effect of psychotherapy: An evaluation". *British Journal of Psychology*, 45, 129–131.

Luborsky, L., Singer, B., & Luborsky, L. (1975). Comparative studies of psychotherapies. Is it true that "everyone has won and all must have prizes". *Archives of General Psychiatry*, 32, 995–1008.

Maslow, A. (1968). *Toward a Psychology of Being*. New York: Van Nostrand.

Metcalfe, J., & Finn, B. (2011). People's hypercorrection of high-confidence errors: Did they know it all along? *Journal of Experimental Psychology: Learning, Memory, and Cognition*, 37, 437–448.

Miller, S.D., Duncan, B.L., Brown, J., Sparks, J., & Claud, D. (2003). The Outcome Rating Scale: A preliminary study of the reliability, validity, and feasibility of a brief visual analog measure. *Journal of Brief Therapy*, 2, 91–100.

Najavits, L.M., & Strupp, H.H. (1994). Differences in the effectiveness of psychodynamic therapists: A process-outcome study. *Psychotherapy: Theory, Research, Practice, Training*, 31, 114–123.

Newport, C. (2012). *So Good They Can't Ignore You. Why Skills Trump Passion in the Quest for Work You Love*. New York: Business Plus.

Nissen-Lie, H.A., Monsen, J.T., & Rønnestad, M.H. (2010). Therapist predictors of early patient-rated working alliance: A multilevel approach. *Psychotherapy Research*, 20, 627–646.

Nissen-Lie, H.A., Rønnestad, M.H., Høglend, P.A., Havik, O.E., Solbakken, O.A., Stiles, T.C., & Monsen, J.T. (2015). Love yourself as a person, doubt yourself as a therapist? *Clinical Psychology & Psychotherapy*, 24. doi:10.1002/cp.1977.

Okiishi, J.C., Lambert, M.J., Nielsen, S.L., & Ogles, B.M. (2003). Waiting for Supershrink: An empirical analysis of therapist effects. *Clinical Psychology and Psychotherapy*, 10, 361–373.

Orlinsky, D.E., & Rønnestad, M.H. (2005). *How Psychotherapists Develop. A Study of Therapeutic Work and Professional Growth*. Washington, DC: American Psychological Association.

Orlinsky, D.E., Rønnestad, M.H., & Willutzki, U. (2004). Fifty Years of Psychotherapy Process-Outcome Research: Continuity and Change. In

M.J. Lambert (Ed.), *Bergin and Garfield's Handbook of Psychotherapy and Behavior Change* (5th ed.). New York: Wiley.

Pink, D.H. (2009). *Drive: The Surprising Truth about What Motivates Us*. New York: Riverhead Books.

Prescott, D.S., Maeschalck, C.L., & Miller, S.D. (Eds.) (2017). *Feedback-Informed Treatment in Clinical Practice: Reaching for Excellence*, Washington, DC: American Psychological Association.

Read, J. (2007). Why promoting biological ideology increases prejudice against people labelled "schizophrenic". *Australian Psychologist*, 42, 118–128.

Reese, R.J., Norsworthy, L.A., & Rowlands, S.R. (2009). Does a continuous feedback system improve psychotherapy outcome? *Psychotherapy Theory, Research, Practice, Training*, 46, 418–431.

Robertson, D.C., & Breen, B. (2013). *Brick by Brick. How LEGO Rewrote the Rules of Innovation and Conquered the Global Toy Industry*. New York: Crown Business.

Rosenzweig, S. (1936). Some implicit common factors in diverse methods of psychotherapy: "At last the Dodo said, 'everyone has won and all must have prizes'". *American Journal of Orthopsychiatry*, 6, 412–415.

Schomerus, G., Schwahn, C., Holzinger, A., Corrigan, P.W., Grabe, H.J., Carta, M.G., & Angermeyer, M.C. (2012). Evolution of public attitudes about mental illness: A systematic review and meta-analysis. *Acta Psychiatrica Scandinavica*, 125, 440–452.

Schultz, H., & Yang, D.J. (1997). *Pour Your Heart into It: How Starbucks Built a Company One Cup at a Time*. New York: Hyperion.

Schulz, K. (2010). *Being Wrong. Adventures in the Margin of Error*. London: Portobello Books.

Schumacher, E.F. (1973). *Small Is Beautiful. A Study of Economics as If People Mattered*. London: Vintage Books.

Schwartz, B., & Sharpe, K. (2010). *Practical Wisdom. The Right Way to Do the Right Thing*. New York: Riverhead Books.

Sims, P. (2011). *Little Bets. How Breakthrough Ideas Emerge from Small Discoveries*. New York: Free Press.

Sinek, S. (2009). *Start with Why. How Great Leaders Inspire Everyone to Take Action*. New York: Portfolio Penguin.

Sirolli, E. (1999). *Ripples from the Zambezi: Passion, Entrepreneurship, and the Rebirth of Local Economies*. Gabriola Island, British Columbia, Canada: New Society Publishers.

Smith, M.L., & Glass, G.V. (1977). Meta-analysis of psychotherapy outcome studies. *American Psychologist*, 32, 752–760.

Snow, C.P. (2001). *De to Kulturer.* Oslo: Cappelen Akademisk.

Stordalen, P. (2009). *Jordbær loso*. Retrieved from http://petterstordalen.no/2009/07/02/jordbærloso/#innhold.

Sundet, R., & Johansen, A. (2012). *Bruken av KOR-skjemaer i "Familiehjelpa i Stange": en forskningsbasert evaluering*. Drammen: IFPR - Institutt for forskning innen psykisk helse og rus, fakultet for helsevitenskap, Høgskolen i Buskerud.

Szasz, T.S. (1974). *The Myth of Mental Illness: Foundations of a Theory of Personal Conduct*. New York: HarperCollins Publishers, Inc.

Tømmerås, S. (2004). Schizofren psychiatri. *Dagbladet*, 15 April 2004.

Tømmerås, S. (2010). Når terapien skader. *Tidsskri for Norsk Psykologforening*, 47, 965.

Ulvestad, A.K., Henriksen, A.K., Tuseth, A., & Fjeldstad, T. (2007). *Klienten – Den Glemte Terapeut. Brukerstyring I Psykisk Helsearbeid*. Oslo: Gyldendal Akademisk.

Valla, B. (2010). Brukers Medvirkning i Psykoterapi – Behov for Kompetanseutvikling. *Tidsskri for Norsk Psykologforening*, 47, 308–314.

Walfish, S., McAlister, B., O'Donnell, P., & Lambert, M.J. (2012). An investigation of self-assessment bias in mental health providers. *Psychological Reports*, 110, 639–644.

Wampold, B.E. (2001). *The Great Psychotherapy Debate. Models, Methods, and Findings*. Mahwah, NJ: Lawrence Erlbaum Associates.

Watkins, C.E. (2010). Psychotherapy supervision since 1909: Some friendly observations about its first century. *Journal of Contemporary Psychotherapy*, 41(2), 57–67.

Watkins, C.E. (2011). Does psychotherapy supervision contribute to patient outcomes? Considering thirty years of research. *The Clinical Supervisor*, 30, 235–256.

Watters, E. (2010). *Crazy Like Us. The Globalization of the American Psyche*. New York: Free Press.

Whitaker, R. (2010). *Anatomy of an Epidemic*. New York: Broadway Paperbacks.

Wiseman, R. (2003). *The Luck Factor.* London: Arrow Books.

INDEX

For Product Safety Concerns and Information please contact our EU
representative GPSR@taylorandfrancis.com
Taylor & Francis Verlag GmbH, Kaufingerstraße 24, 80331 München, Germany

www.ingramcontent.com/pod-product-compliance
Ingram Content Group UK Ltd.
Pitfield, Milton Keynes, MK11 3LW, UK
UKHW022201190926
475702UK00003B/151
9780367175108